Upper Gastrointestinal Malignancies

Editor

MANISH A. SHAH

HEMATOLOGY/ONCOLOGY CLINICS OF NORTH AMERICA

www.hemonc.theclinics.com

Consulting Editors
GEORGE P. CANELLOS
H. FRANKLIN BUNN

June 2017 • Volume 31 • Number 3

ELSEVIER

1600 John F. Kennedy Boulevard • Suite 1800 • Philadelphia, Pennsylvania, 19103-2899

http://www.theclinics.com

HEMATOLOGY/ONCOLOGY CLINICS OF NORTH AMERICA Volume 31, Number 3
June 2017 ISSN 0889-8588, ISBN 13: 978-0-323-53011-8

Editor: Stacy Eastman
Developmental Editor: Kristen Helm

Hematology/Oncology Clinics (ISSN 0889-8588) is published bimonthly by Elsevier Inc., 360 Park Avenue South, New York, NY 10010-1710. Months of issue are February, April, June, August, October, and December. Business and Editorial Offices: 1600 John F. Kennedy Blvd., Ste. 1800, Philadelphia, PA 19103—2899. Customer Service Office: 3251 Riverport Lane, Maryland Heights, MO 63043. Periodicals postage paid at New York, NY and at additional mailing offices. Subscription prices are $397.00 per year (domestic individuals), $742.00 per year (domestic institutions), $100.00 per year (domestic students/residents), $453.00 per year (Canadian individuals), $919.00 per year (Canadian institutions) $536.00 per year (international individuals), $919.00 per year (international institutions), and $255.00 per year (international and Canadian students/residents). International air speed delivery is included in all *Clinics* subscription prices. All prices are subject to change without notice. **POSTMASTER:** Send address changes to *Hematology/Oncology Clinics of North America*, Elsevier Health Sciences Division, Subscription Customer Service, 3251 Riverport Lane, Maryland Heights, MO 63043. Customer Service (orders, claims, online, change of address): Elsevier Health Sciences Division, Subscription **Customer Service, 3251 Riverport Lane, Maryland Heights, MO 63043. Tel: 1-800-654-2452 (U.S. and Canada); 314-447-8871 (outside U.S. and Canada). Fax: 314-447-8029. E-mail: journalscustomerservice-usa@elsevier.com (for print support); journalsonlinesupport-usa@elsevier.com (for online support).**

Reprints. For copies of 100 or more, of articles in this publication, please contact the Commercial Reprints Department, Elsevier Inc., 360 Park Avenue South, New York, New York 10010-1710; Tel.: 212-633-3874, Fax: 212-633-3820, E-mail: reprints@elsevier.com.

Hematology/Oncology Clinics of North America is covered in *MEDLINE/PubMed (Index Medicus), EMBASE/ Excerpta Medica, and BIOSIS.*

Contributors

CONSULTING EDITORS

GEORGE P. CANELLOS, MD
William Rosenberg Professor of Medicine, Department of Medical Oncology, Dana-Farber Cancer Institute, Boston, Massachusetts

H. FRANKLIN BUNN, MD
Professor of Medicine, Division of Hematology, Brigham and Women's Hospital, Harvard Medical School, Boston, Massachusetts

EDITOR

MANISH A. SHAH, MD
Division of Hematology and Medical Oncology, Department of Medicine, Weill Cornell Medical College of Cornell University, Bartlett Family Associate Professor of Gastrointestinal Oncology, Director, Gastrointestinal Oncology Program, Co-Director, Center for Advanced Digestive Care, Sandra and Edward Meyer Cancer Center, Associate Professor, New York-Presbyterian Hospital, Weill Cornell Medicine, New York, New York

AUTHORS

SALAH-EDDIN AL-BATRAN, MD
Professor, Institute of Clinical Cancer Research, Krankenhaus Nordwest, UCT-University Cancer Center, Frankfurt am Main, Germany

WILLIAM ALLUM, MD
Departments of Gastrointestinal Oncology, Radiology, and Surgery, Royal Marsden Hospital, London, United Kingdom

GAYATHRI ANANDAPPA, MBBS, MRCP(UK), MPhil(Cantab)
Clinical Research Fellow, Department of Medicine, Royal Marsden Hospital, London, United Kingdom; Department of Medicine, Royal Marsden Hospital, Surrey, United Kingdom

DORON BETEL, PhD
Assistant Professor of Computational Biomedicine, Institute for Computational Biomedicine, Co-Director of the Epigenomics Core Facility, Division of Hematology and Medical Oncology, Department of Medicine, Weill Cornell Medical College of Cornell University, New York, New York

DANIEL V.T. CATENACCI, MD
Associate Director, Gastrointestinal Oncology Program, Assistant Professor of Medicine, Section of Hematology/Oncology, University of Chicago Comprehensive Cancer Center, Chicago, Illinois

IAN CHAU, MBBS, FRCP(UK), MD
Consultant Oncologist, Department of Medicine, Royal Marsden Hospital, London, United Kingdom; Department of Medicine, Royal Marsden Hospital, Surrey, United Kingdom

THOMAS HAYES, MB ChB
Departments of Gastrointestinal Oncology, Radiology, and Surgery, Royal Marsden Hospital, London, United Kingdom

ZHAOHUI JIN, MD
Department of Medical Oncology, Mayo Clinic, Rochester, Minnesota

RONAN J. KELLY, MB, BCh, MBA
Director of the Gastro-esophageal Cancer Therapeutics Program, Upper Aerodigestive Malignancies Division, The Sidney Kimmel Comprehensive Cancer Center, Johns Hopkins Medicine, Baltimore, Maryland

PERCY LEE, MD
Associate Professor, Department of Radiation Oncology, Jonsson Comprehensive Cancer Center, David Geffen School of Medicine, University of California Los Angeles, Los Angeles, California

FLORIAN LORDICK, MD, PhD
Professor and Director, University Cancer Center Leipzig (UCCL), University Hospital Leipzig, Leipzig, Germany

SYLVIE LORENZEN, MD
Department of Hematology and Oncology, Klinikum rechts der Isar, Technical University (TU), München, München, Germany

STEVEN B. MARON, MD
Fellow, Section of Hematology/Oncology, University of Chicago Comprehensive Cancer Center, Chicago, Illinois

ADRIAN G. MURPHY, MB, BCh, PhD
Gastrointestinal Malignancies Division, The Sidney Kimmel Comprehensive Cancer Center, Johns Hopkins Medicine, Baltimore, Maryland

JOHN NG, MD
Assistant Professor, Department of Radiation Oncology, Weill Cornell Medical College, New York-Presbyterian Hospital, New York, New York

RADKA OBERMANNOVÁ, MD, PhD
Assistant Professor and Consulting Physician, Clinic of Comprehensive Cancer Care, Masaryk Memorial Cancer Institute, Faculty of Medicine, Masaryk University, Brno, Czech Republic

SARAH ELLEN POWELL, PhD
Division of Hematology and Medical Oncology, Department of Medicine, Weill Cornell Medical College of Cornell University, New York, New York

SHANMUGARAJAH RAJENDRA, MSc, MD, FRACP
Gastro-Intestinal Viral Oncology Group, Ingham Institute for Applied Medical Research, South Western Sydney Clinical School, University of New South Wales, Department of Gastroenterology & Hepatology, Bankstown-Lidcombe Hospital, South Western Sydney Local Health Network, Sydney, New South Wales, Australia

ANGELA RIDDELL, MD
Departments of Gastrointestinal Oncology, Radiology, and Surgery, Royal Marsden Hospital, London, United Kingdom

MANISH A. SHAH, MD
Division of Hematology and Medical Oncology, Department of Medicine, Weill Cornell Medical College of Cornell University, Bartlett Family Associate Professor of Gastrointestinal Oncology, Director, Gastrointestinal Oncology Program, Co-Director, Center for Advanced Digestive Care, Sandra and Edward Meyer Cancer Center, Associate Professor, New York-Presbyterian Hospital, Weill Cornell Medicine, New York, New York

PRATEEK SHARMA, MD, FACG
Division of Gastroenterology and Hepatology, Veterans Affairs Medical Center, University of Kansas School of Medicine, Kansas City, Missouri

ELIZABETH SMYTH, MB BCh, MSc
Departments of Gastrointestinal Oncology, Radiology, and Surgery, Royal Marsden Hospital, London, United Kingdom

HARRY H. YOON, MD, MHS
Assistant Professor of Oncology, Department of Medical Oncology, Mayo Clinic, Rochester, Minnesota

CHAO ZHANG, PhD
Institute for Computational Biomedicine, Division of Hematology and Medical Oncology, Department of Medicine, Weill Cornell Medical College of Cornell University, New York, New York

Contents

Tumor Biology

> Gastric malignancies are a leading cause of cancer-related death world-
> wide. At least 2 microbial species are currently linked to carcinogenesis
> and the development of cancer within the human stomach. These include
> the bacterium *Helicobacter pylori* and the Epstein-Barr virus. In recent
> years, there has been increasing evidence that within the human gastroin-
> testinal tract it is not only pathogenic microbes that impact human health
> but also the corresponding autochthonous microbial communities. This
> article reviews the gastrointestinal microbiome as it relates primarily to
> mechanisms of disease and carcinogenesis within the upper gastrointes-
> tinal tract.

> Barrett esophagus (BE) is a precursor lesion for esophageal adenocarci-
> noma (EAC). Developments in imaging and molecular markers, and endo-
> scopic eradication therapy, are available to curb the increase of EAC.
> Endoscopic surveillance is recommended, despite lack of data. The can-
> cer risk gets progressively downgraded, raising questions about the un-
> derstanding of risk factors and molecular biology involved. Recent data
> point to at least 2 carcinogenic pathways operating in EAC. The use of
> p53 overexpression and high-risk human papillomavirus may represent
> the best chance to detect progressors. Genome-wide technology may
> provide molecular signatures to aid diagnosis and risk stratification in BE.

Management

> Gastric and esophageal tumors have a poor prognosis; approximately
> 15% of patients are alive at 10 years following diagnosis. Surgical resec-
> tion plus adjunctive chemotherapy or chemoradiotherapy is curative in
> approximately 50% of patients with operable disease, but is also associ-
> ated with significant morbidity. Therefore, accurate preoperative staging
> is required to spare patients unnecessary toxicity and futile surgery. This
> review evaluates the sensitivity and specificities of the modalities used
> to stage patients with gastroesophageal cancer. Staging techniques

success of immune checkpoint inhibitors in other tumor types, for example, lung cancer and melanoma, much attention is being paid to furthering their role in gastric and esophageal cancers. The Cancer Genome Atlas has provided further details of the molecular heterogeneity of these tumors, which may help predict responsiveness to immune checkpoint inhibitors. This article discusses the rationale for investigating these agents in gastroesophageal cancer and summarizes the relevant clinical trial data and ongoing studies.

Antiangiogenesis therapy is one of only 2 biologically targeted approaches shown to improve overall survival over standard of care in advanced adenocarcinoma of the stomach or gastroesophageal junction (GEJ). Therapeutic targeting of vascular endothelial growth factor receptor 2 improves overall survival in patients with previously treated advanced gastric/GEJ adenocarcinoma. No antiangiogenesis therapy has demonstrated an overall survival benefit in patients with chemo-naïve or resectable esophagogastric cancer or in patients whose tumors arise from the esophagus. Promising ongoing clinical investigations include the combination of antiangiogenesis therapy with immune checkpoint inhibition and anti–human epidermal growth factor receptor 2 therapy.

Gastroesophageal cancer (GEC) remains a major cause of cancer-related mortality worldwide. Although the incidence of distal gastric adenocarcinoma (GC) is declining in the United States, proximal esophagogastric junction adenocarcinoma (EGJ) incidence is rising. GC and EGJ, together, are treated uniformly in the metastatic setting as GEC. Overall survival in the metastatic setting remains poor, with few molecular targeted approaches having been successfully incorporated into routine care to date—only first-line anti-HER2 therapy for *ERBB2* amplification and second-line anti-VEGFR2 therapy. This article reviews aberrations in epidermal growth factor receptor, *MET,* and *ERBB2,* their therapeutic implications, and future directions in targeting these pathways.

With further understanding of the biology of gastric and gastroesophageal adenocarcinomas, strides are being made to find effective treatments through novel trial designs. This article focuses on the ongoing trials of drugs targeting specific hallmarks of gastric and gastroesophageal cancers, including oncogene addiction proliferative pathways (fibroblast growth factor receptor 2 amplified tumors), stem cell inhibition, apoptotic induction through claudin inhibitors, and matrix metalloproteinase inhibition. In developing novel therapeutics in treatment of patients with gastroesophageal adenocarcinomas, parallel research efforts to refine target population and biomarkers are crucial, and targeting the tumor genomics and microenvironment may be key in improving overall survival.

This issue of *Hematology/Oncology Clinics of North America* provides an update to the current understanding of the physiology of gastric and esophageal cancers and the state-of-the-art management of disease. Over the past 10 years, we have witnessed dramatic changes in both our understanding of the disease and its management. We have 2 new biological agents approved to treat advanced disease, with several more prospects under development. In this article, the author looks to the future, attempting to answer the question of which advancements will play the biggest role in improving patient outcomes in this still-devastating disease.

HEMATOLOGY/ONCOLOGY CLINICS OF NORTH AMERICA

THE CLINICS ARE AVAILABLE ONLINE!
Access your subscription at:
www.theclinics.com

Preface

The Management of Esophagogastric Cancers Enters a New Era

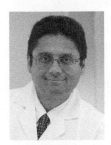

Manish A. Shah, MD
Editor

This timely issue of *Hematology/Oncology Clinics of North America* highlights the current management of cancers of the foregut (esophagus and stomach). Cancers of the esophagus and stomach remain prevalent, and together, are more common globally than cancers of the colon and rectum or hepatocellular cancer. Importantly, these cancers still carry a poor prognosis and remain a fruitful area for research and drug development. I am very proud of this issue and in particular of my friends and colleagues who were able to contribute scholarly articles that help define the disease and our care. In this issue, we highlight the current understanding of disease biology and epidemiology, including the potential impact of the microbiome on carcinogenesis. We also address current concepts in cancer staging and management of localized disease. For more advanced disease, it is important to understand that we have witnessed an explosion of novel treatments for solid tumor malignancies, including therapies that augment the immune response to tumors. In cancers of the esophagus and stomach, we have been able to add novel targeted agents to our armamentarium of cytotoxic therapies, including agents that target angiogenesis and the epidermal growth factor pathway. However, most impressive is that there are currently thousands of patients with foregut malignancies that are enrolled in clinical trials examining novel treatment strategies and novel therapeutics. This explosion of activity will be accompanied by many new treatment options for our patients moving forward. Herein, we provide a context of standard treatment options as well as novel therapies that appear promising. Although, unfortunately, most patients with cancers of the esophagus and stomach will ultimately die of their disease, there is tremendous hope that we are in the dawn of a new era in the management of these diseases: where understanding the biology and carcinogenesis of the disease will lead to smarter ways to prevent or screen for the disease, where management of localized disease will have more specific

Hematol Oncol Clin N Am 31 (2017) xiii–xiv
http://dx.doi.org/10.1016/j.hoc.2017.03.001
0889-8588/17/© 2017 Published by Elsevier Inc.

hemonc.theclinics.com

and targeted algorithms, and where new treatments will be identified that can dramatically improve upon or augment the outcomes we observe with chemotherapy alone. I enjoin you to continue reading and contribute to this transformation that I see coming for patients with gastric and esophageal cancer.

Manish A. Shah, MD
Gastrointestinal Oncology Program
Center for Advanced Digestive Care
Sandra and Edward Meyer Cancer Center
at Weill Cornell Medicine
1305 York Avenue, 12th Floor
New York, NY 10021, USA

E-mail address:
mas9313@med.cornell.edu

Tumor Biology

The Gastric Microbiome and Its Influence on Gastric Carcinogenesis
Current Knowledge and Ongoing Research

Chao Zhang, PhD[a,b], Sarah Ellen Powell, PhD[b], Doron Betel, PhD[a,b], Manish A. Shah, MD[b,c],*

KEYWORDS

- Gastric microbiome • *Helicobacter pylori* • EBV • Gastric cancer
- Microbial identification

KEY POINTS

- Gastric cancer is the fourth leading cause of cancer-related deaths worldwide, most commonly caused by chronic infection with intracellular bacterium *Helicobacter pylori*.
- *H pylori* is the most common cause of peptic ulcer disease. The drivers that determine malignant transformation over self-limiting ulcer and chronic gastritis remain unknown.
- In addition to *H pylori*, the stomach hosts a diverse and active microbial community whose role in host response and pathogenesis has yet to be fully delineated.
- The gastric microbiome is likely a marker of host health and influences the inflammatory response within upper gastrointestinal cancers.

INTRODUCTION

The human body is thought to house more than 100 trillion microbes. These microbial communities have a significant impact on their human hosts.[1] They influence everything from pathogen defense to digestion to immune system maturation. The microbiome is also linked to the development of several autoimmune diseases and cancers, including colorectal, pancreatic, and gastric cancers.[2] A major risk factor for the development of gastric cancer (GC) is infection by the bacteria *Helicobacter*

[a] Institute for Computational Biomedicine, Weill Cornell Medicine, New York, NY 10021, USA; [b] Division of Hematology and Medical Oncology, Department of Medicine, Weill Cornell Medicine, New York, NY 10021, USA; [c] Gastrointestinal Oncology Program, Center for Advanced Digestive Care, Sandra and Edward Meyer Cancer Center, New York-Presbyterian Hospital, Weill Cornell Medicine, New York, NY 10021, USA
* Corresponding author. Division of Hematology and Medical Oncology, New York-Presbyterian Hospital, Weill Cornell Medicine, 1305 York Avenue, Room Y1247, New York, NY 10021.
E-mail address: mas9313@med.cornell.edu

Hematol Oncol Clin N Am 31 (2017) 389–408
http://dx.doi.org/10.1016/j.hoc.2017.01.002
0889-8588/17/© 2017 Elsevier Inc. All rights reserved.

pylori, a common inhabitant (although not always pathogen) of the human stomach. GC is the fourth most common cancer worldwide. The study of *H pylori* and its associated gastric microbiome is of increasing importance in the study of gastrointestinal (GI) diseases and chronic immune response. Understanding the impact of microbial community structure and function on tumorigenesis and immune response will broaden the understanding of GC tumorigenesis and may impact development of therapeutic and preventative approaches.

MICROBIOME DIVERSITY ALONG THE GASTROINTESTINAL TRACT

Although parts of the GI tract are arguably primed for microbial life, the stomach is not intuitively such an environment. The human stomach is particularly unique in that its inhabitants are challenged by several antimicrobial chemicals, enzymes, structural barriers, and highly acidic conditions that are not collectively present in any other part of the human body. Although transient microbes may temporarily survive such an environment through spore formation, thickened cell walls, and acid resistance, those colonizing this environment must adapt to a highly variable and ever-changing landscape.

A benefit of the harsh gastric environment is that it enables segregation of digestive absorption of food from most of the microbial biomass, thereby prioritizing nutrient absorption. The production of salivary enzymes such as lipase and amylase as well as the conversion of nitrates into the antimicrobial compound NO_2 by *Lactobacilli* in the mouth begins the process of dramatically reducing the microbial biomass before microbial entry into the stomach.[3] Microbes entering the stomach are then exposed to hydrochloric acid secreted by parietal cells, which then enables the conversion of pepsinogen into pepsin, a potent enzyme that denatures proteins and inhibits microbial survival and growth.

In addition to antimicrobial enzymes, there are several other mechanisms used by the host to prevent microbial proliferation within the stomach. Antimicrobial mechanisms include the expression of immunoglobulin A (IgA), which is thought to limit mucosal penetration and potentially shape diversity of normal gut flora.[4] In addition, the constitutive production of defensins and cathelicidins in epithelial cells as well as triggered expression of C-type lectins help to protect host mucosa from over colonization.[5]

These challenges largely explain the discordance in the bacterial density in the stomach as compared with the colon. By some estimates, microbial cell numbers increase from 10^1 to 10^3 colony-forming units (CFU) mL^{-1} in the stomach to 10^{11}–10^{12} cfu mL^{-1} in the large intestine. Notably, the colonic bacterial density exceeds that found in any other known ecosystem.[5,6]

Gastric Bacteria

Bacteria that are able to reside in the stomach demonstrate several mechanisms that enable colonization within the harsh gastric environment. Acid resistance is a significant factor for bacterial survival and proliferation. Bacteria such as *Escherichia coli* and *H pylori* exhibit increased membrane protein production and buffering capacity, allowing these bacteria to resist acid degradation upon entry to the stomach. Subsequent structural, enzymatic, and adhesive adaptive advantages further enable these bacteria and others to colonize the environment.[7,8]

Multiple studies have attempted to characterize the microbial components of the stomach, either directly from biopsy samples or from gastric juices. There is increasing evidence that the microbiome profiles of the human stomach vary widely between individuals with some consistency as to common phyla, although not necessarily species. The most dominant bacterial phyla found across multiple studies are Proteobacteria, Firmicutes, Actinobacteria, and Bacteroidetes[9–14] (**Table 1**). Several studies also mention frequency of the phyla Fusobacteria.[10,15–17] Numerous other phyla have also been detected in lower abundance across gastric samples.

Prevalent species consistent across multiple studies included *Streptococcus* sp, *Lactobacillus* sp, *Veillonella* sp, *Prevotella* sp, *Rothia* sp, and *Neisseria* sp (see **Table 1**). More than 65% of the phylotypes of bacteria found in the stomach are also those known to inhabit the human mouth[3] (**Fig. 1**).

More than 260 microbial phylotypes have been isolated from as few as 3 separate gastric samples, with only 33 phyla shared between them.[15] Gall and colleagues[19] demonstrated that bacterial communities in the upper GI tract displayed higher interindividual variation but overlapping community membership between anatomic sites, indicating that a single set of microbiome profiles of the gastric environment is not generalizable nor directly applicable to any one individual (see **Fig. 1**). This study also found that samples from the same individual were more likely to be phylogenetically similar to each other than to samples from the same anatomic site in other individuals.[19]

Bacterial composition and diversity seem to also depend on other species cohabiting the gut. Ecologically, many bacteria rely on commensal, syntrophic, and symbiotic relationships, and this is often reflected in community structure and diversity. For example, *H pylori* is known to reduce the acidity within the stomach, thus enabling other bacteria to colonize an environment where they might not otherwise survive. Therefore, the representation of dominant phyla in the stomach between the *H pylori*–positive and –negative profiles is notably different. In one study, up to 28% of total variance in gastric microbiota between subjects was explained by *H pylori* infection status.[12]

Esophageal Bacteria

Biopsies from the normal human esophagus commonly contain bacterial members of the phyla Firmicutes, Bacteroides, Actinobacteria, Proteobacteria, and Fusobacteria.[20] Although the predominant phyla of the esophagus fit the profile of those found within the gastric environment, the species composition is fundamentally different.

Table 1
Common genera and phyla of the gastric microbiome (*Helicobacter pylori* excluded)

Genera	Gram +/−	Phylum	Relative Abundance, %
Bifidobacteria sp[15,17]	POS	Actinobacteria	10.7–46.8
Rothia sp[10,15]	POS		
Prevotella sp[10,11,15–17]	NEG	Bacteroidetes	11.1–26
Enterococcus sp[14,17]	POS	Firmicutes	29.6–51
Gemella sp[15,17]	POS		
Lactobacillus sp[9,13,14,16–18]	POS		
Streptococcus sp[9–11,14–18]	POS		
Staphylococcus sp[9,13,14,18]	POS		
Veillonella sp[9,10,16]	POS		
Fusobacterium sp[10,17]	NEG	Fusobacteria	<1.1
Campylobacter sp[14,17]	NEG	Proteobacteria	6.9–10.8
Haemophilus sp[9,11,17]	NEG		
Neisseria sp[9,11,17,18]	NEG		

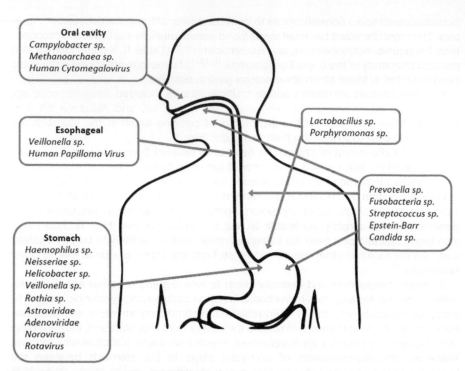

Oral cavity
Campylobacter sp.
Methanoarchaea sp.
Human Cytomegalovirus

Esophageal
Veillonella sp.
Human Papilloma Virus

Lactobacillus sp.
Porphyromonas sp.

Prevotella sp.
Fusobacteria sp.
Streptococcus sp.
Epstein-Barr
Candida sp.

Stomach
Haemophilus sp.
Neisseriae sp.
Helicobacter sp.
Veillonella sp.
Rothia sp.
Astroviridae
Adenoviridae
Norovirus
Rotavirus

Fig. 1. Common species in upper GI tract.

Streptococcus sp comprised almost 40% of bacterial composition, whereas *Prevotella* sp and *Veilonella* sp were 17% and 14%, respectively. In one study, up to 87% of bacteria were shared between normal tissues from patients, indicating that the esophagus may house a less diverse population of bacteria between individuals than the stomach.[20]

A more detailed set of studies investigating esophageal microbiota demonstrated at least 2 distinct microbiome profiles distinguish healthy normal esophageal tissue from gastroesophageal reflux disease (GERD) patients. The profile associated with normal tissue was dominated by *Streptococcus* sp and en mass contained predominantly gram-positive bacteria belonging to the Firmicutes phyla. The profile most associated with esophagitis and GERD contained primarily gram-negative, anaerobic, or microaerophilic bacteria and a dominance of Bacteroidetes, Proteobacteria, Spirochaetes, and Fusobacteria phyla, respectively. Changes in relative abundance of these taxa appear to play a more significant role than absolute bacterial loads.[21]

Viruses

Viruses as autochthonous, nonpathogenic inhabitants of the human gastric environment have not been widely studied. To date, there are few known benign viral inhabitants of the stomach. Those known to cause severe gastritis, such as Norovirus, Rotavirus, Astroviridae, and Adenoviridae, are temporary infections generally cleared by the host immune system after a short infectious course. A significant viral pathogen associated with the development of a genetically distinct GC subtype is Epstein-Barr virus (EBV),[22] described in detail later in this review. Human papilloma virus has been strongly correlated with esophageal squamous carcinoma and may play a mechanistic role for the development of other cancers along the GI tract.[23] Other oncogenic viruses infecting other regions of the body that may yet be found to influence the gastric environment include human cytomegalovirus, Merkel cell polycomavirus, and hepatitis B and C viruses.[24,25] When combined statistically to those cancers caused by *H pylori* bacterium, these microbial pathogens may account for more than 15% of the cancer burden worldwide.[26]

Archaea

Archaea are single-celled prokaryotic organisms that are members of their own genetically distinct domain. They are notorious extremophiles. Found in geothermal vents, miles beneath the surface of the ocean, and even in volcanoes, this group consists of many organisms primed for otherwise inhospitable conditions.[27]

The human gut is host to several archaea, notably methane-producing species known as methanogens. Two main species frequently inhabit the gut: *Methanobrevibacter smithii* and *Methanosphaera stadtmanae* (MSS), likely metabolically supporting surrounding bacterial communities.[28] Although few studies to date have attempted to elucidate archaea from the stomach specifically, it is highly likely given their ecology that these microbes are found in abundance throughout the GI tract.

Methanoarchaea are frequently able to form syntrophic interactions with a wide range of bacterial constituents, and in some cases, are necessary for their survival, metabolic function, and growth.[29] For some beneficial bacteria, they are necessary cohabitants of the environment. They possess metabolic processes that convert common bacterial fermentation byproducts such as hydrogen and carbon dioxide and enable interspecies hydrogen transfer.[30] Studies of archaea composition within patients with cancer suffering from chemotherapy-induced diarrhea demonstrated a decrease of methanogenic archaea in parallel with the loss of beneficial bacteria.[31]

Despite ubiquitous distribution and high numbers within the human gut, archaea have not generally been recognized as significant components of the microbiota and the immune system. Associations between *Methanobrevibacter oralis* and inflammatory periodontal disease have, however, led to further interest in the potential pathogenic potential of some archaea.[32,33]

Blais Lecours and colleagues[34] found increased prevalence of MSS in patients with inflammatory bowel disease (IBD). Only IBD patients developed a significant anti-MSS IgG response.[34] Additional evidence suggests methane production by archaea is related to pathogenesis of constipation, irritable bowel syndrome (IBS), and obesity. Many patients with IBS and constipation excrete methane, suggesting an overabundance of methanogenic archaea in their gut.[35] In a more recent study, differences in archaea and microbial composition were observed in colorectal tubular adenoma and adenocarcinoma cases between both healthy and diseased mucosa.[36] It is apparent from such studies that archaea have the potential to influence both community structure within the microbiome and immune response. As such, they should not be overlooked.

Fungi

Fungi are a ubiquitous but often ignored component of the gastric microbiome. Surveys of the gastric environment identified hundreds of diverse fungal strains, including representatives from *Candida albicans*, *Candida tropicales*, and *Candida lusitanae* within both the healthy gut and those with GI ulcers. Fungi survive much higher acidities than many bacteria due to structural and biological adaptations. *C albicans* are able to proliferate at a pH of 1.4 and upwards. Comparative studies of fungi colonizing gastric ulcers found 54.2% of cases had fungal infections compared with 10.3% of those with chronic gastritis and 4.3% of controls. Measurements of antifungal antibodies and the presence of fungal antigens within these study subjects' serum indicated that fungal colonizations were likely secondary features of other infections; however, they are likely still important in the context of the gastric microbial milieu.[37]

IDENTIFICATION METHODOLOGIES FROM CLINICAL SAMPLES
Experimental Approaches

Studying microbes within the gastric environment is particularly challenging given the low abundance and the lack of ability to culture these organisms. More than 80% of microbes are uncultivable.[3]

Even with well-established culture independent methods such as the isolation and amplification of 16S ribosomal RNA (rRNA) genes by polymerase chain reaction (PCR) and quantitative PCR, microbial DNA isolation from human tissue is notoriously subject to bias. The bias of 16S-based methods often results from environmental conditions and the ability of extraction techniques to account for natural differences in microbial cell wall structure as well as susceptibility of certain microbial species to lysis. Bacteria in particular may exhibit varying levels of resistance to release their nucleic acids using chaotropic agents, enzymes, homogenization, or bead-beating.[38] As such, there is not a single "gold standard" by which to determine environmental composition of human samples. Several methods are described in the literature to try to address this disparity with varying results in terms of diversity, species selection, and abundance.[39,40] For any extractions intended for downstream sequencing, it is therefore important to be aware that extraction methodologies may not capture the full spectrum of bacterial composition of the samples.

Some other culture-independent methods used to obtain an accurate profile of these microbes include fluorescent in situ hybridization, dot-blot hybridization with rRNA-targeted probes, denaturing gradient gel electrophoresis, cloning, and more recently, whole genome shotgun (WGS) sequencing.[38] Although no method is immune to bias, analyses like whole genome sequencing enable a much more sensitive means to obtain microbial sequences and data. Using additional computational pipelines, it is possible to achieve another lens with which to view the microbial constituents of the human microbiome.

Computational Identification of Microbiome

The computational approaches to identify the microbiome have been specifically designed to process 16S rRNA gene or WGS sequencing, respectively. The bacterial and archaeal 16S rRNA gene has been widely used as the phylogenetic marker for microbial characterization due to its universal presence in prokaryotes. Several different taxonomic schemes have been proposed by independent curators based on structural and functional attributes of microbes, and 16S rRNA sequences, for example, Berpey's,[41] National Center for Biotechnology Information. All major rRNA gene sequence databases, such as RDP,[42] Greengenes,[43] and SILVA,[44] were designed based on different taxonomic schemes and accumulated vast reference sequences for phylogenetic analysis. Generally, algorithms for microbial identification from 16S rRNA data can be divided into 2 major categories: homology based and composition based.[45] Homology-based approaches use traditional sequence alignment algorithms to compare similarity between sequencing data and reference 16S rRNA in the database. Composition-based methods build models based on the different features extracted from sequences, for example, GC content, codon usage, and frequencies of motifs. To date, most microbiome studies rely on 16S rRNA-based method, because it is cost-effective, and data processing is easier than WGS data. The limitation of this method is that the taxonomic annotation is based on putative association of one single gene. In practice, only 1 of 2 variable regions of 16S rRNA is amplified. Because of its highly conserved nature, typically it only analyzes at the phyla or genus level, and identification at the species level could be less accurate. For example, different species within the same genus, such as Bacillus cereus, Bacillus thuringiensis, and Bacillus anthracis,[46] have only a few base differences in their 16S rRNA gene sequences.

As the alternative approach, WGS appears to be more accurate to profile the microbiome to species level, even to subspecies level, but it is more expensive and requires extensive data analysis. Computational methods to identify microbes from WGS can generally be classified, similarly to 16S, as homology based and composition based. A potential limitation of WGS is that most algorithms require complete genomes to build databases in order to achieve precision. Although a recent publication partially addressed this problem by constructing the database with detected clade-specific markers,[47] it sacrifices the identification accuracy to reduce the computational complexity. Unlike 16S rRNA genes that are specific to prokaryotes, WGS sequencing approach captures host DNA as well. The relative abundance of host contamination is as high as 99.9% in human clinical biopsies. Although a pipeline with extensive filtering steps that maps sequencing reads to different human sequence databases could remove most host content,[48] the remaining reads may still lead to false identification within traditional microbiome profiling software, which is designed to process microbial DNA-enriched samples.[14] Thus, additional steps are necessary to accurately characterize microbial species for host DNA-enriched samples, such as genome coverage evaluation.[14]

A myriad of factors can affect microbial detection, including different experiment protocols, different reference databases, different species markers, and different mapping algorithms. Although it is unlikely that different identification approaches will agree in bacterial identification, the most abundant species should always be detected by all methods.

EPIDEMIOLOGIC ASSOCIATIONS WITH DISEASES
Helicobacter pylori

GC is a heterogeneous disease with several established risk factors, one of the most significant being chronic gastric inflammation due to infection by the gram-negative, facultative intracellular bacillus H pylori.[49]

Unlike other common factors causing acute gastritis, H pylori–associated acute gastritis is usually asymptomatic[50]; thus, it could be easily ignored and delayed. Several studies show strong correlations between H pylori and acute gastritis. Harford and colleagues[51] performed a long-term follow-up study on 35 cases of acute gastritis with hypochlorhydria. Twenty-eight of 35 participants either had a positive H pylori infection history or had a new infection within 12 months. Cheung and colleagues[52] completed gastroscopies for 194 participants out of a population of 600 from Aklavik, Canada. Among 128 participants who were histologically H pylori positive, prevalence was 94% for acute gastritis and 100% for chronic gastritis.

After persistent colonization within the gastric mucosa, H pylori has been significantly associated with the development of different stages of gastric diseases, from chronic gastritis,[53,54] gastric ulcers,[55,56] atrophic gastritis,[57,58] intestinal metaplasia,[59,60] and finally, to GC.[61–63] Several studies and meta-analyses support these findings.

Besides gastritis and GC, H pylori has also been identified as a risk factor for other upper GI diseases. The study by Eidt and colleagues[64] found that nearly all patients with gastric mucosa-associated lymphoid tissue lymphoma are *H pylori* positive. Although there are multiple factors that may cause functional dyspepsia, *H pylori* is still considered a likely culprit.[65,66] A recent retrospective study of 5156 patients revealed that *H pylori* infection was significantly more common among those with GERD (odds ratio = 1.17).[67] Interestingly, *H pylori* also has been reported with inverse correlations to some diseases. Multiple meta-analyses revealed that decline of *H pylori* colonization in the past few decades may be responsible for an increase of esophageal cancer incidence in Western countries.[68,69] Although 95% duodenal ulcer occurred in the presence of *H pylori* infection,[56] in the cohort of patients with duodenal ulcers, the incidence of GC was significantly lower than expected.[70]

Epstein-Barr Virus

As another identified risk factor for developing GC, EBV[71] is responsible for 5% to 20% of GC worldwide. Global infection prevalence of EBV is approximately 9%, which is much lower than that of *H pylori*. Only a small proportion of GC is associated with EBV infection; therefore, most epidemiologic studies cannot find strong correlations due to the limited data.[72] Although EBV has been suspected in several other upper GI diseases, most studies to date are only case reports,[73,74] and a lack of large-scale studies cannot currently support the causal relationships between EBV and these diseases.

Other

Because of a lack of understanding of the gastric microbiome as a whole, most epidemiologic studies are limited to *H pylori* and EBV.[75] Only a few studies have looked at the community of bacteria and their overall relationship to GC. Aviles-Jimenez and colleagues[76] found a significant microbial difference between nonatrophic gastritis (NAG) and intestinal-type GC. *Porphyromonas*, *Neisseria*, TM7 group, and *Streptococcus sinensis* decrease, whereas *Lactobacillus coleohominis* and Lachnospiraceae increase from NAG to GC. Seo and colleagues[77] evaluated cancer tissue and matching normal gastric mucosa from 16 patients. According to the genus level comparison, they found that *Propionibacterium* spp, *Staphylococcus* spp, and *Corynebacterium* spp had significantly reduced populations in cancer tissue, whereas *Clostridium* spp and *Prevotella* spp had significantly increased populations. Eun and colleagues[78] used 454 sequencing to sequence the V5 region of 16S rDNA from 31 patients. They found that compared with chronic gastritis and intestinal metaplasia groups, the relative abundance of Bacilli class and Streptococcaceae families increased, and the Helicobacteraceae family was significantly lower in GC group.

MOLECULAR ASSOCIATIONS AND MECHANISMS OF TUMORIGENESIS

Bacteria within the human body produce low molecular weight substances that, although difficult to isolate, are attributable to epigenetic changes. The epigenetic changes include chromatin remodeling and signaling molecule changes, which regulate cellular differentiation and apoptosis as well as inflammation.[79] These changes may also lead to tumorigenesis. The mechanisms behind these relationships are complex and may have larger implications for the study of oncogenic potential among several bacteria found within the human microbiome.

Mechanisms of Helicobacter pylori Tumorigenicity

H pylori invades and damages the gastric mucosa using a series of competitive mechanisms specifically adapted to colonize the gastric environment. The major mechanisms include structural and adhesive advantages such as flagella that enable motility and penetration of the gastric mucin layer. *H pylori* binds to mucin and targets gastric epithelial cells. Its flagella are protected by a lipopolysaccharides-containing sheath and protein, which generate an immune response mediating mucous synthesis and secretion by epithelial cells.[80,81] Another colonizing advantage of *H pylori* is the production of urease enzyme. Urease produces ammonia from urea, thereby neutralizing nitric acid within the stomach and allowing access to the mucus layer. *H pylori* is then able to colonize the epithelium and elicit an intricate immune response of inflammatory cytokines leading to peptic ulcers or chronic gastritis.[3]

Highly carcinogenic strains of *H pylori* carry the cytotoxin-associated gene A (cagA). This gene encodes for CagA, a known regulator of malignancy. Bacterial type IV secretions deliver CagA into gastric epithelial cells.[82] CagA disrupts host signaling pathways by acting as a hub or extrinsic scaffold protein, in turn potentiating genomic instability or malignant transformation.[83,84]

Transgenic mice who systemically express wild-type CagA have been known to spontaneously develop GI carcinomas, whereas phosphorylation-resistant CagA fails to induce such malignancy.[85] CagA is stabilized through phosphorylation, which in turn enables binding to SHP2 and subsequent activation of the Ras-Erk mitogenic pathway.[86] Genes often overexpressed in GC are involved in this signaling pathway. The Ras-Erk mitogenic pathway include FGFR2, KRAS, EGFR, ERBB2, and MET, which are frequently investigated targets for drug treatment.[87–89] Overexpression of above genes leads to unique DNA damage in transcribed regions and those proximal to telomeres in gastric cell lines and primary gastric epithelial cells.[90]

In addition to CagA, several other bacterial virulence factors play a role in both the pathogenisis and the inflammatory potential of *H pylori*. These virulence factors include Vacuolating cytotoxin A and its associated polymorphisms as well as outer membrane proteins BabA, HomA, and HomB.[91] HomB in Western-type CagA strains have been directly associated with the development of GC.[92]

The interactions between *H pylori* and other microbiota within the gastric environment are complex and are mediated in part by host response. *H pylori* uses BabA and Cag plasminogen activator inhibitor proteins to adhere to epithelial cells, which promotes expression of inflammatory cytokines, including IL-1b, IL-6, IL-8, and IL-10, as well as tumor necrosis factor-α, exacerbating immune responses.[93–95] Immune exacerbation in turn likely impacts the success of other bacterial species. *H pylori* also affects the hormones and density-dependent humoral and cellular immune responses within the gastric environment.[96,97] Hormones that modulate immunity and gastric acid secretion promote a Th1 response.[98,99] More research is needed to characterize the physiologic differences related to *H pylori* status, including variation in the gastric microbiota, as well as its clinical implications.[12]

EVIDENCE FOR PROLONGED MICROBIOME SHIFTS ASSOCIATED WITH PRIOR INFECTION WITH *HELICOBACTER PYLORI*

Another unique feature of *H pylori* infection within the gut is its potential for long-term disturbances of the microbiota even after individuals clear infection. A recent study examining the stool of patients previously infected with *H pylori* found that up to 18 months after eradication there is still a disruption in the phyla and genera of microbes seen within the lower GI tract. Yap and colleagues[100] found a continual increase in Firmicutes and decrease in Bacteroidetes species at 6 months, 12 months, and 18 months after infection, respectively. Bacteroidetes and Firmicutes are associated with the regulation of lipids and bile acid metabolic processes. Disturbances in these balances have been implicated in metabolic disorders and obesity.[101] Long-term perturbations of the gut microbiota due to *H pylori* infection may therefore have further implications for host immune response and recovery.

Epstein-Barr Virus

EBV-associated gastric carcinoma (EBVaGC) is a distinct subtype that has very distinguished molecular characteristics compared with other GC subtypes defined by The Cancer Genome Atlas study.[102] Although some of the molecular mechanisms underlying EBVaGC are still unclear, several studies have already demonstrated the genomic features of EBVaGC. These studies provide an important understanding of EBV involvement in gastric carcinogenesis.[103–105]

Latent infection in gastric epithelial cells

Previous studies reveal that EBV can readily infect B lymphocytes through viral receptor CD21. Because epithelial cells lack the expression of CD21, the efficiency of EBV infection is much lower.[106] Coculturing epithelial cells with EBV-producing B-lymphoblastoid cells will significantly increase infection efficiency,[107] and direct cell-to-cell contact with B lymphocytes might be the major model of EBV infection within epithelial cells.[103] After infection is established in epithelial cells, EBV will maintain a latent infection status and only express a limited set of viral genes, such as EBERs, EBNA-1, and BARTs. The functions of these viral genes were investigated in several studies[108–111] and were found to have interactions with host proteins that affect cell proliferation, apoptosis resistance, and production of autocrine growth factors. The resulting DNA damage and promotion of cell survival contribute to the development of GC.

Epigenetic alterations

Besides direct manipulating cell proliferation and migration, EBV also can disrupt host epigenetic machinery to affect the host epigenome on its path to malignancy.[112] EBVaGC exhibits the global but nonrandom CpG island hypermethylation at various tumor suppressor genes such as PTEN. By expressing LMP1 and LMP2A viral oncoproteins to upregulate host DNMTs,[110] EBV not only can inactivate these host tumor suppressors but also may have its own DNA methylated to evade host immune response.[113] However, the target specificity for these processes remains unclear. Different studies have reported several sets of genes that are hypermethylated in EBVaGC rather than other GC subtypes, but there is no single gene present in all 3 major studies on the topic.[102,114,115]

Viral microRNAs

The EBV genome encodes 25 microRNA (miRNA) precursors and 44 mature miRNAs. Among them, only 22 miRNA precursors from BART cluster are expressed in EBVaGC.[116] Several studies revealed that a set of EBV miRNAs, ebv-miR-BART1-3p, 2-5p, 3, 4, 5, 7, 9, 10-3p, 17-5p, and 18-5p, were expressed at relatively high levels in EBVaGC, and some of them could target the tumor suppressor gene PTEN.[117] They also observed the downregulation of human cellular miRNAs, such as hsa-miR-200a, hsa-miR-200b, and let-7 family, which are tumor suppressor miRNAs.[116] Viral miRNA involvement in EBVaGC remains largely unknown. Besides regulating the gene expression, viral miRNAs might also interfere with intercellular communication and modify the tumor microenvironment.[118] EBV miRNAs could be transferred from EBV-infected cells to noninfected cells through exosome transfer,[119] and they accumulate in noninfected cells to induce apoptosis in Jurkat T cells.[120]

Mechanisms of Fusobacterium sp

In addition to *H pylori*, another gastric bacterium that has recently been identified as significantly oncogenic is *Fusobacterium nucleatum. Fusobacterium* sp are gram-negative, non-spore-forming, anaerobic bacteria that are commonly isolated bacterial flora throughout the human GI tract. The species *F nucelatum*, however, is associated with several other disease manifestations such as periodontitis as well as tumor growth and carcinogenesis of both pancreatic and colorectal cancer.[121–123] Colorectal carcinoma tissue has also been shown to frequently be enriched by this bacterium.[124] More recently, *F nucleatum* positivity has been linked to microsatellite instability (MSI-high) and CpG island methylator phenotype status in studies involving large US and Japanese colorectal cancer cohorts.[125] MSI and other molecular characteristics of colorectal cancer influence T-cell-mediated adaptive immunity. Mechanistically, *F nucleatum* in colorectal tumors appears to have the capacity to expand myeloid-derived immune cells and inhibit T-cell proliferation, inducing T-cell apoptosis.[125] As such, this bacterium may prove to have more serious immune implications in other regions of the GI tract, such as the stomach, and its impact on the gastric microenvironment has yet to be thoroughly investigated.

Other Species

Given the relatively recent discovery of *H pylori* and *F nucleatum* as known gastric bacteria with tumorigenic potential, it is likely that with improved surveillance and additional focus on the microbiome as an indicator for immune health, there are several other microbes with significant tumorigenic mechanisms yet to be fully elucidated in the gastric environment.

Several bacterial species are also coming to light with regard to gut-derived cancers that may be connected to the stomach microbiota as well. Retrospective studies have shown associations between *Streptococcus* sp and both oral and colorectal cancer, whereas *Salmonella typhi* has shown capacity for the manipulation of host signaling pathways leading to gallbladder carcinomas, respectively.[126–128] *Streptococcus* species are frequently isolated within the stomach, and their carcinogenic potential therein has not yet been fully explored.

Notable temporal and spatial links between periodontal disease–causing bacteria and oral and esophageal cancers have also recently emerged, begging the question whether this association also may extend to microbial inhabitants of the stomach and other carcinogenic mechanisms throughout the body. *H pylori* and *Fusobacterium* have already been isolated from periodontal pockets, sometimes forming biofilms and coaggregating to form dental plaques.[129] The relationship between this co-occurrence and further infection potential within the greater GI tract has yet to be fully understood.

Chronic inflammation caused by other orally derived species, such as *Campylobacter concisus, Porphyromonas gigivalis,* and *Prevotella melaninogenica,* has been linked to periodontal lesions as well as increased expression of biomarkers and cytokines for carcinogenesis, potentially promoting the development of esophageal and oral cancers as well as some cases of pancreatic cancer.[127,130] These relationships will likely only prove more important as we continue to build on the understanding of oral microbiota and the spatial and temporal relationships between inflammation and immune response throughout the GI tract.

"COMMUNITY AS PATHOGEN"—COMMUNITY DYNAMICS AND PATHOBIONTS

The microbiome as a whole is defined as the sum total genome of all bacteria, archaea, fungi, protozoa, and viruses inhabiting the human body[75] (see **Fig. 1**). In many ways, these communities are analogous to isolated ecosystems with defined trophic architecture, ecological niches, and community assemblages that determine overall environmental health and stability. Much as a rainforest or reef system experiences disturbances, community assemblage overturn, and invasive species, which may alter entire species composition and ultimate homeostasis of a given environment, so too might this occur within the gut. Rather than identifying single pathogens as the causative agent for chronic inflammation and tumorigenesis, it is becoming increasingly evident that several environmental and community factors often come into play to potentiate these effects. These factors include conditions promoted by pathogenic symbionts or "pathobionts" of otherwise commensal bacteria within the human gut.[131] When, for example, H pylori lowers the acidity profile of the gastric environment, it is an ecological disturbance that in turn affects community structure and perhaps the ability for pathobionts to proliferate and impact other aspects of host health (**Fig. 2**). This ecological disturbance could be observed within the esophageal environment as well. Unlike gastric malignancies, which have been correlated to specific infections by EBV or H pylori, GERD, esophageal adenocarcinomas, and other malignancies have been attributed to chronically disrupted microbiome profiles and dysbiosis.[132]

Microbial profile variations as well as community interdependence between and within individuals may offer valuable clues to the origins of cancer development,

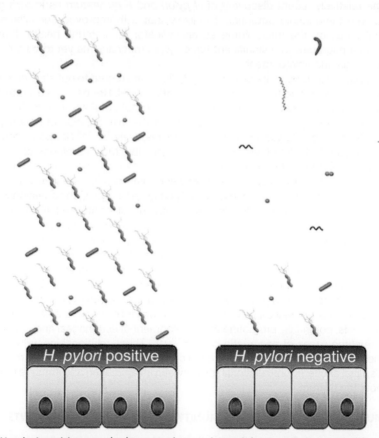

Fig. 2. H pylori–positive samples have much more bacterial contents than negative samples, but are also less diverse.

disease prognosis, and immune system health. Current evidence that the microbiome may be linked to immunotherapy response within the colon and infections with *H pylori* leads to long-term perturbations of gut stability further illustrates the importance of understanding these relationships.[100] Preliminary studies have shown positive correlations between abundance of certain commensal gut bacteria within the colon and antitumor responses. Specifically, colonization by various *Bifidobacterium* sp has demonstrated an improved response to anti-PDL1 therapy.[133] However, precisely what effect a given homeostasis or biodiversity may have on chronic inflammation, immune status, and several other factors on the human body has yet to be fully understood.

CHALLENGES AND ONGOING RESEARCH

Gastric microbiota is strongly associated with many upper GI diseases, including cancer. *H pylori* itself is estimated to contribute to 5.5% of all cancer cases and more than 60% of GC cases.[26] Gastric microbiota is still ignored by most GC studies, because stomach has been considered a sterile environment for a very long period. Hebert and colleagues[134] revealed that only less than 10% National Cancer Institute–supported grants for GC research incorporated microbiome analysis, indicating lack of attention toward gastric microbiome study. Among all *H pylori*–infected individuals, only 1% to 3% develop GC.[135] Gastric tumorigenesis studies should incorporate host genetic characteristic and virulence diversity of *H pylori* strains as well as the entire microbiome community. Notably, GC development might take longer than 20 years, and ideal design of the study should include long-term observations on microbiome dynamics and spontaneous host genetic changes over the time, such as mutation accumulation.

REFERENCES

1. Gill SR, Pop M, Deboy RT, et al. Metagenomic analysis of the human distal gut microbiome. Science 2006;312(5778):1355-9.
2. Fujimura KE, Slusher NA, Cabana MD, et al. Role of the gut microbiota in defining human health. Expert Rev Anti Infect Ther 2010;8(4):435-54.
3. Nardone G, Compare D. The human gastric microbiota: is it time to rethink the pathogenesis of stomach diseases? United Eur Gastroenterol J 2015;3(3): 255-60.
4. Suzuki K, Meek B, Doi Y, et al. Aberrant expansion of segmented filamentous bacteria in IgA-deficient gut. Proc Natl Acad Sci U S A 2004;101(7):1981-6.
5. Walter J, Ley R. The human gut microbiome: ecology and recent evolutionary changes. Annu Rev Microbiol 2011;65:411-29.
6. Eckburg PB, Bik EM, Bernstein CN, et al. Diversity of the human intestinal microbial flora. Science 2005;308(5728):1635-8.
7. Mobley HLT, Mendz GL, Hazell SL, editors. Helicobacter pylori: physiology and genetics. Washington, DC: ASM Press; 2001.
8. Booth IR. Regulation of cytoplasmic pH in bacteria. Microbiol Rev 1985;49(4): 359-78.
9. Mowat C, Williams C, Gillen D, et al. Omeprazole, Helicobacter pylori status, and alterations in the intragastric milieu facilitating bacterial N-nitrosation. Gastroenterology 2000;119(2):339-47.
10. Bik EM, Eckburg PB, Gill SR, et al. Molecular analysis of the bacterial microbiota in the human stomach. Proc Natl Acad Sci U S A 2006;103(3):732-7.

11. Li XX, Wong GL, To KF, et al. Bacterial microbiota profiling in gastritis without Helicobacter pylori infection or non-steroidal anti-inflammatory drug use. PLoS One 2009;4(11):e7985.

12. Maldonado-Contreras A, Goldfarb KC, Godoy-Vitorino F, et al. Structure of the human gastric bacterial community in relation to Helicobacter pylori status. ISME J 2011;5(4):574–9.

13. Hu Y, He LH, Xiao D, et al. Bacterial flora concurrent with Helicobacter pylori in the stomach of patients with upper gastrointestinal diseases. World J Gastroenterol 2012;18(11):1257–61.

14. Zhang C, Cleveland K, Schnoll-Sussman F, et al. Identification of low abundance microbiome in clinical samples using whole genome sequencing. Genome Biol 2015;16:265.

15. Andersson AF, Lindberg M, Jakobsson H, et al. Comparative analysis of human gut microbiota by barcoded pyrosequencing. PLoS One 2008;3(7):e2836.

16. Dicksved J, Lindberg M, Rosenquist M, et al. Molecular characterization of the stomach microbiota in patients with gastric cancer and in controls. J Med Microbiol 2009;58(Pt 4):509–16.

17. von Rosenvinge EC, Song Y, White JR, et al. Immune status, antibiotic medication and pH are associated with changes in the stomach fluid microbiota. ISME J 2013;7(7):1354–66.

18. Kato S, Fujimura S, Kimura K, et al. Non-Helicobacter bacterial flora rarely develops in the gastric mucosal layer of children. Dig Dis Sci 2006;51(4):641–6.

19. Gall A, Fero J, McCoy C, et al. Bacterial composition of the human upper gastrointestinal tract microbiome is dynamic and associated with genomic instability in a Barrett's esophagus cohort. PLoS One 2015;10(6):e0129055.

20. Pei Z, Bini EJ, Yang L, et al. Bacterial biota in the human distal esophagus. Proc Natl Acad Sci U S A 2004;101(12):4250–5.

21. Yang L, Lu X, Nossa CW, et al. Inflammation and intestinal metaplasia of the distal esophagus are associated with alterations in the microbiome. Gastroenterology 2009;137(2):588–97.

22. Iizasa H, Nanbo A, Nishikawa J, et al. Epstein-Barr virus (EBV)-associated gastric carcinoma. Viruses 2012;4(12):3420–39.

23. Ding GC, Ren JL, Chang FB, et al. Human papillomavirus DNA and P16(INK4A) expression in concurrent esophageal and gastric cardia cancers. World J Gastroenterol 2010;16(46):5901–6.

24. Feng H, Shuda M, Chang Y, et al. Clonal integration of a polyomavirus in human Merkel cell carcinoma. Science 2008;319(5866):1096–100.

25. Mesri EA, Feitelson MA, Munger K. Human viral oncogenesis: a cancer hallmarks analysis. Cell Host Microbe 2014;15(3):266–82.

26. Parkin DM. The global health burden of infection-associated cancers in the year 2002. Int J Cancer 2006;118(12):3030–44.

27. Bang C, Schmitz RA. Archaea associated with human surfaces: not to be underestimated. FEMS Microbiol Rev 2015;39(5):631–48.

28. Dridi B, Henry M, El Khechine A, et al. High prevalence of Methanobrevibacter smithii and Methanosphaera stadtmanae detected in the human gut using an improved DNA detection protocol. PLoS One 2009;4(9):e7063.

29. Samuel BS, Gordon JI. A humanized gnotobiotic mouse model of host-archaeal-bacterial mutualism. Proc Natl Acad Sci U S A 2006;103(26):10011–6.

30. Thauer RK, Shima S. Biogeochemistry: methane and microbes. Nature 2006; 440(7086):878–9.

31. Stringer AM, Al-Dasooqi N, Bowen JM, et al. Biomarkers of chemotherapy-induced diarrhoea: a clinical study of intestinal microbiome alterations, inflammation and circulating matrix metalloproteinases. Support Care Cancer 2013; 21(7):1843–52.

32. Lepp PW, Brinig MM, Ouverney CC, et al. Methanogenic archaea and human periodontal disease. Proc Natl Acad Sci U S A 2004;101(16):6176–81.

33. Vianna ME, Holtgraewe S, Seyfarth I, et al. Quantitative analysis of three hydrogenotrophic microbial groups, methanogenic archaea, sulfate-reducing bacteria, and acetogenic bacteria, within plaque biofilms associated with human periodontal disease. J Bacteriol 2008;190(10):3779–85.

34. Blais Lecours P, Marsolais D, Cormier Y, et al. Increased prevalence of Methanosphaera stadtmanae in inflammatory bowel diseases. PLoS One 2014;9(2): e87734.

35. Pimentel M, Mathur R, Chang C. Gas and the microbiome. Curr Gastroenterol Rep 2013;15(12):356.

36. Mira-Pascual L, Cabrera-Rubio R, Ocon S, et al. Microbial mucosal colonic shifts associated with the development of colorectal cancer reveal the presence of different bacterial and archaeal biomarkers. J Gastroenterol 2015;50(2):167–79.

37. Zwolinska-Wcislo M, Budak A, Bogdal J, et al. Fungal colonization of gastric mucosa and its clinical relevance. Med Sci Monit 2001;7(5):982–8.

38. Sheh A, Fox JG. The role of the gastrointestinal microbiome in Helicobacter pylori pathogenesis. Gut Microbes 2013;4(6):505–31.

39. Yuan S, Cohen DB, Ravel J, et al. Evaluation of methods for the extraction and purification of DNA from the human microbiome. PLoS One 2012;7(3):e33865.

40. Ó Cuív P, Aguirre de Carcer D, Jones M, et al. The effects from DNA extraction methods on the evaluation of microbial diversity associated with human colonic tissue. Microb Ecol 2011;61(2):353–62.

41. Vos P, Garrity G, Jones D, et al. Bergey's manual of systematic bacteriology: volume 3: the firmicutes, vol. 3. New York: Springer Science & Business Media; 2011.

42. Cole JR, Wang Q, Fish JA, et al. Ribosomal database project: data and tools for high throughput rRNA analysis. Nucleic Acids Res 2014;42(Database issue): D633–42.

43. DeSantis TZ, Hugenholtz P, Larsen N, et al. Greengenes, a chimera-checked 16S rRNA gene database and workbench compatible with ARB. Appl Environ Microbiol 2006;72(7):5069–72.

44. Pruesse E, Quast C, Knittel K, et al. SILVA: a comprehensive online resource for quality checked and aligned ribosomal RNA sequence data compatible with ARB. Nucleic Acids Res 2007;35(21):7188–96.

45. Zhang C, Zheng G, Xu S-F, et al. Computational challenges in characterization of bacteria and bacteria-host interactions based on genomic data. J Computer Sci Technology 2012;27(2):225–39.

46. Sacchi CT, Whitney AM, Mayer LW, et al. Sequencing of 16S rRNA gene: a rapid tool for identification of Bacillus anthracis. Emerg Infect Dis 2002;8(10):1117–23.

47. Segata N, Waldron L, Ballarini A, et al. Metagenomic microbial community profiling using unique clade-specific marker genes. Nat Methods 2012;9(8): 811–4.

48. Kostic AD, Ojesina AI, Pedamallu CS, et al. PathSeq: software to identify or discover microbes by deep sequencing of human tissue. Nat Biotechnol 2011;29(5):393–6.

49. Brawner KM, Morrow CD, Smith PD. Gastric microbiome and gastric cancer. Cancer J 2014;20(3):211–6.

50. Sugano K, Tack J, Kuipers EJ, et al. Kyoto global consensus report on Helicobacter pylori gastritis. Gut 2015;64(9):1353–67.

51. Harford WV, Barnett C, Lee E, et al. Acute gastritis with hypochlorhydria: report of 35 cases with long term follow up. Gut 2000;47(4):467–72.

52. Cheung J, Goodman KJ, Girgis S, et al. Disease manifestations of Helicobacter pylori infection in Arctic Canada: using epidemiology to address community concerns. BMJ Open 2014;4(1). e003689.

53. Basso D, Plebani M, Kusters JG. Pathogenesis of Helicobacter pylori infection. Helicobacter 2010;15(Suppl 1):14–20.

54. Watari J, Chen N, Amenta PS, et al. Helicobacter pylori associated chronic gastritis, clinical syndromes, precancerous lesions, and pathogenesis of gastric cancer development. World J Gastroenterol 2014;20(18):5461–73.

55. Nomura A, Stemmermann GN, Chyou PH, et al. Helicobacter pylori infection and the risk for duodenal and gastric ulceration. Ann Intern Med 1994;120(12): 977–81.

56. Kuipers EJ, Thijs JC, Festen HP. The prevalence of Helicobacter pylori in peptic ulcer disease. Aliment Pharmacol Ther 1995;9(Suppl 2):59–69.

57. Kamada T, Haruma K, Ito M, et al. Time trends in helicobacter pylori infection and atrophic gastritis over 40 years in Japan. Helicobacter 2015;20(3):192–8.

58. Joo YE, Park HK, Myung DS, et al. Prevalence and risk factors of atrophic gastritis and intestinal metaplasia: a nationwide multicenter prospective study in Korea. Gut Liver 2013;7(3):303–10.

59. Peleteiro B, Lunet N, Figueiredo C, et al. Smoking, Helicobacter pylori virulence, and type of intestinal metaplasia in Portuguese males. Cancer Epidemiol Biomarkers Prev 2007;16(2):322–6.

60. Park YH, Kim N. Review of atrophic gastritis and intestinal metaplasia as a premalignant lesion of gastric cancer. J Cancer Prev 2015;20(1):25–40.

61. Chen XZ, Schottker B, Castro FA, et al. Association of helicobacter pylori infection and chronic atrophic gastritis with risk of colonic, pancreatic and gastric cancer: a ten-year follow-up of the ESTHER cohort study. Oncotarget 2016; 7(13):17182–93.

62. Lee YC, Chen TH, Chiu HM, et al. The benefit of mass eradication of Helicobacter pylori infection: a community-based study of gastric cancer prevention. Gut 2013;62(5):676–82.

63. Huang JQ, Zheng GF, Sumanac K, et al. Meta-analysis of the relationship between cagA seropositivity and gastric cancer. Gastroenterology 2003;125(6): 1636–44.

64. Eidt S, Stolte M, Fischer R. Helicobacter pylori gastritis and primary gastric non-Hodgkin's lymphomas. J Clin Pathol 1994;47(5):436–9.

65. Talley NJ, Ford AC. Functional dyspepsia. N Engl J Med 2015;373(19):1853–63.

66. Rokkas T. The role of Helicobacter pylori infection in functional dyspepsia. Ann Gastroenterol 2012;25(2):176–7.

67. Dore MP, Pes GM, Bassotti G, et al. Risk factors for erosive and non-erosive gastroesophageal reflux disease and Barrett's esophagus in Nothern Sardinia. Scand J Gastroenterol 2016;51(11):1281–7.

68. Islami F, Kamangar F. Helicobacter pylori and esophageal cancer risk: a meta-analysis. Cancer Prev Res (Phila) 2008;1(5):329–38.

69. Thrift AP, Pandeya N, Smith KJ, et al. Helicobacter pylori infection and the risks of Barrett's oesophagus: a population-based case-control study. Int J Cancer 2012;130(10):2407–16.
70. Hansson LE, Nyren O, Hsing AW, et al. The risk of stomach cancer in patients with gastric or duodenal ulcer disease. N Engl J Med 1996;335(4):242–9.
71. Boyle P, Levin B. World cancer report 2008. Lyon, France: IARC Press, International Agency for Research on Cancer; 2008.
72. Kelley JR, Duggan JM. Gastric cancer epidemiology and risk factors. J Clin Epidemiol 2003;56(1):1–9.
73. Hisamatsu A, Nagai T, Okawara H, et al. Gastritis associated with Epstein-Barr virus infection. Intern Med 2010;49(19):2101–5.
74. Owens SR, Walls A, Krasinskas AM, et al. Epstein-Barr virus gastritis: rare or rarely sampled? A case report. Int J Surg Pathol 2011;19(2):196–8.
75. Vogtmann E, Goedert JJ. Epidemiologic studies of the human microbiome and cancer. Br J Cancer 2016;114(3):237–42.
76. Aviles-Jimenez F, Vazquez-Jimenez F, Medrano-Guzman R, et al. Stomach microbiota composition varies between patients with non-atrophic gastritis and patients with intestinal type of gastric cancer. Sci Rep 2014;4:4202.
77. Seo I, Jha BK, Suh S-I, et al. Microbial profile of the stomach: comparison between normal mucosa and cancer tissue in the same patient. J Bacteriol Virol 2014;44(2):162–9.
78. Eun CS, Kim BK, Han DS, et al. Differences in gastric mucosal microbiota profiling in patients with chronic gastritis, intestinal metaplasia, and gastric cancer using pyrosequencing methods. Helicobacter 2014;19(6):407–16.
79. Paul B, Barnes S, Demark-Wahnefried W, et al. Influences of diet and the gut microbiome on epigenetic modulation in cancer and other diseases. Clin Epigenetics 2015;7:112.
80. Testerman TL, McGee DJ, Mobley HLT. Adherence and colonization. In: Mobley HLT, Mendz GL, Hazell SL, editors. Helicobacter pylori: physiology and genetics. Washington, DC: ASM Press; 2001.
81. Zhang C, Xu S, Xu D. Risk assessment of gastric cancer caused by Helicobacter pylori using CagA sequence markers. PLoS One 2012;7(5):e36844.
82. Hatakeyama M. Helicobacter pylori CagA and gastric cancer: a paradigm for hit-and-run carcinogenesis. Cell Host Microbe 2014;15(3):306–16.
83. Higashi H, Tsutsumi R, Fujita A, et al. Biological activity of the Helicobacter pylori virulence factor CagA is determined by variation in the tyrosine phosphorylation sites. Proc Natl Acad Sci U S A 2002;99(22):14428–33.
84. Mueller D, Tegtmeyer N, Brandt S, et al. c-Src and c-Abl kinases control hierarchic phosphorylation and function of the CagA effector protein in Western and East Asian Helicobacter pylori strains. J Clin Invest 2012;122(4):1553–66.
85. Ohnishi N, Yuasa H, Tanaka S, et al. Transgenic expression of Helicobacter pylori CagA induces gastrointestinal and hematopoietic neoplasms in mouse. Proc Natl Acad Sci U S A 2008;105(3):1003–8.
86. Saito Y, Murata-Kamiya N, Hirayama T, et al. Conversion of Helicobacter pylori CagA from senescence inducer to oncogenic driver through polarity-dependent regulation of p21. J Exp Med 2010;207(10):2157–74.
87. Shah MA. Update on metastatic gastric and esophageal cancers. J Clin Oncol 2015;33(16):1760–9.
88. Umeda M, Murata-Kamiya N, Saito Y, et al. Helicobacter pylori CagA causes mitotic impairment and induces chromosomal instability. J Biol Chem 2009; 284(33):22166–72.

89. Luo CH, Chiou PY, Yang CY, et al. Genome, integration, and transduction of a novel temperate phage of Helicobacter pylori. J Virol 2012;86(16):8781–92.

90. Koeppel M, Garcia-Alcalde F, Glowinski F, et al. Helicobacter pylori infection causes characteristic DNA damage patterns in human cells. Cell Rep 2015; 11(11):1703–13.

91. Jones KR, Whitmire JM, Merrell DS. A tale of two toxins: helicobacter pylori CagA and VacA modulate host pathways that impact disease. Front Microbiol 2010;1:115.

92. Talebi Bezmin Abadi A, Rafiei A, Ajami A, et al. Helicobacter pylori homB, but not cagA, is associated with gastric cancer in Iran. J Clin Microbiol 2011; 49(9):3191–7.

93. Atherton JC, Peek RM Jr, Tham KT, et al. Clinical and pathological importance of heterogeneity in vacA, the vacuolating cytotoxin gene of Helicobacter pylori. Gastroenterology 1997;112(1):92–9.

94. Rad R, Gerhard M, Lang R, et al. The Helicobacter pylori blood group antigen-binding adhesin facilitates bacterial colonization and augments a nonspecific immune response. J Immunol 2002;168(6):3033–41.

95. Yamaoka Y, Kita M, Kodama T, et al. Induction of various cytokines and development of severe mucosal inflammation by cagA gene positive Helicobacter pylori strains. Gut 1997;41(4):442–51.

96. Plebani M, Basso D, Cassaro M, et al. Helicobacter pylori serology in patients with chronic gastritis. Am J Gastroenterol 1996;91(5):954–8.

97. Atherton JC, Blaser MJ. Coadaptation of Helicobacter pylori and humans: ancient history, modern implications. J Clin Invest 2009;119(9):2475–87.

98. Faggioni R, Feingold KR, Grunfeld C. Leptin regulation of the immune response and the immunodeficiency of malnutrition. FASEB J 2001;15(14):2565–71.

99. Perry S, de Jong BC, Solnick JV, et al. Infection with Helicobacter pylori is associated with protection against tuberculosis. PLoS One 2010;5(1):e8804.

100. Yap TW, Gan HM, Lee YP, et al. Helicobacter pylori eradication causes perturbation of the human gut microbiome in young adults. PLoS One 2016;11(3): e0151893.

101. Turnbaugh PJ, Ley RE, Mahowald MA, et al. An obesity-associated gut microbiome with increased capacity for energy harvest. Nature 2006;444(7122): 1027–31.

102. Cancer Genome Atlas Research Network. Comprehensive molecular characterization of gastric adenocarcinoma. Nature 2014;513(7517):202–9.

103. Shinozaki-Ushiku A, Kunita A, Fukayama M. Update on Epstein-Barr virus and gastric cancer (review). Int J Oncol 2015;46(4):1421–34.

104. Gulley ML. Genomic assays for Epstein-Barr virus-positive gastric adenocarcinoma. Exp Mol Med 2015;47:e134.

105. Abe H, Kaneda A, Fukayama M. Epstein-Barr virus-associated gastric carcinoma: use of host cell machineries and somatic gene mutations. Pathobiology 2015;82(5):212–23.

106. Tsao SW, Tsang CM, Pang PS, et al. The biology of EBV infection in human epithelial cells. Semin Cancer Biol 2012;22(2):137–43.

107. Imai S, Nishikawa J, Takada K. Cell-to-cell contact as an efficient mode of Epstein-Barr virus infection of diverse human epithelial cells. J Virol 1998; 72(5):4371–8.

108. Chang MS, Kim DH, Roh JK, et al. Epstein-Barr virus-encoded BARF1 promotes proliferation of gastric carcinoma cells through regulation of NF-kappaB. J Virol 2013;87(19):10515–23.

109. Sivachandran N, Dawson CW, Young LS, et al. Contributions of the Epstein-Barr virus EBNA1 protein to gastric carcinoma. J Virol 2012;86(1):60–8.
110. Zhao J, Liang Q, Cheung KF, et al. Genome-wide identification of Epstein-Barr virus-driven promoter methylation profiles of human genes in gastric cancer cells. Cancer 2013;119(2):304–12.
111. Banerjee AS, Pal AD, Banerjee S. Epstein-Barr virus-encoded small non-coding RNAs induce cancer cell chemoresistance and migration. Virology 2013;443(2): 294–305.
112. Birdwell CE, Queen KJ, Kilgore PC, et al. Genome-wide DNA methylation as an epigenetic consequence of Epstein-Barr virus infection of immortalized keratino- cytes. J Virol 2014;88(19):11442–58.
113. Hino R, Uozaki H, Murakami N, et al. Activation of DNA methyltransferase 1 by EBV latent membrane protein 2A leads to promoter hypermethylation of PTEN gene in gastric carcinoma. Cancer Res 2009;69(7):2766–74.
114. Matsusaka K, Kaneda A, Nagae G, et al. Classification of Epstein-Barr virus- positive gastric cancers by definition of DNA methylation epigenotypes. Cancer Res 2011;71(23):7187–97.
115. Wang K, Yuen ST, Xu J, et al. Whole-genome sequencing and comprehensive molecular profiling identify new driver mutations in gastric cancer. Nat Genet 2014;46(6):573–82.
116. Marquitz AR, Mathur A, Chugh PE, et al. Expression profile of microRNAs in Epstein-Barr virus-infected AGS gastric carcinoma cells. J Virol 2014;88(2): 1389–93.
117. Cai LM, Lyu XM, Luo WR, et al. EBV-miR-BART7-3p promotes the EMT and metastasis of nasopharyngeal carcinoma cells by suppressing the tumor sup- pressor PTEN. Oncogene 2015;34(17):2156–66.
118. Pegtel DM, van de Garde MD, Middeldorp JM. Viral miRNAs exploiting the endosomal-exosomal pathway for intercellular cross-talk and immune evasion. Biochim Biophys Acta 2011;1809(11–12):715–21.
119. Pegtel DM, Cosmopoulos K, Thorley-Lawson DA, et al. Functional delivery of viral miRNAs via exosomes. Proc Natl Acad Sci U S A 2010;107(14):6328–33.
120. Qu JL, Qu XJ, Qu JL, et al. The role of cbl family of ubiquitin ligases in gastric cancer exosome-induced apoptosis of Jurkat T cells. Acta Oncol 2009;48(8): 1173–80.
121. Signat B, Roques C, Poulet P, et al. Fusobacterium nucleatum in periodontal health and disease. Curr Issues Mol Biol 2011;13(2):25–36.
122. Castellarin M, Warren RL, Freeman JD, et al. Fusobacterium nucleatum infection is prevalent in human colorectal carcinoma. Genome Res 2012;22(2):299–306.
123. Mitsuhashi K, Nosho K, Sukawa Y, et al. Association of Fusobacterium species in pancreatic cancer tissues with molecular features and prognosis. Oncotarget 2015;6(9):7209–20.
124. Mima K, Sukawa Y, Nishihara R, et al. Fusobacterium nucleatum and T cells in colorectal carcinoma. JAMA Oncol 2015;1(5):653–61.
125. Nosho K, Sukawa Y, Adachi Y, et al. Association of Fusobacterium nucleatum with immunity and molecular alterations in colorectal cancer. World J Gastroen- terol 2016;22(2):557–66.
126. Gold JS, Bayar S, Salem RR. Association of Streptococcus bovis bacteremia with colonic neoplasia and extracolonic malignancy. Arch Surg 2004;139(7): 760–5.
127. Chocolatewala N, Chaturvedi P, Desale R. The role of bacteria in oral cancer. In- dian J Med Paediatr Oncol 2010;31(4):126–31.

128. Scanu T, Spaapen RM, Bakker JM, et al. Salmonella manipulation of host signaling pathways provokes cellular transformation associated with gall-bladder carcinoma. Cell Host Microbe 2015;17(6):763–74.

129. Al Asqah M, Al Hamoudi N, Anil S, et al. Is the presence of Helicobacter pylori in dental plaque of patients with chronic periodontitis a risk factor for gastric infection? Can J Gastroenterol 2009;23(3):177–9.

130. Hajishengallis E, Parsaei Y, Klein MI, et al. Advances in the microbial etiology and pathogenesis of early childhood caries. Mol Oral Microbiol 2017;32(1): 24–34.

131. Chow J, Tang H, Mazmanian SK. Pathobionts of the gastrointestinal microbiota and inflammatory disease. Curr Opin Immunol 2011;23(4):473–80.

132. Pei Z, Yang L, Peek RM Jr, et al. Bacterial biota in reflux esophagitis and Barrett's esophagus. World J Gastroenterol 2005;11(46):7277–83.

133. Sivan A, Corrales L, Hubert N, et al. Commensal Bifidobacterium promotes anti-tumor immunity and facilitates anti-PD-L1 efficacy. Science 2015;350(6264): 1084–9.

134. Hebert EF, Divi RL, Verma M. Microbiome analysis: trends in cancer epidemiology, challenges and opportunities. Int J Cancer Res Mol Mech 2015;1(1).

135. Peek RM Jr, Crabtree JE. Helicobacter infection and gastric neoplasia. J Pathol 2006;208(2):233–48.

Barrett Esophagus and Intramucosal Esophageal Adenocarcinoma

 CrossMark

Shanmugarajah Rajendra, MSc, MD, FRACP[a,b,*],
Prateek Sharma, MD[c]

KEYWORDS

- Barrett esophagus • Esophageal adenocarcinoma • Human papillomavirus
- Screening • Surveillance

KEY POINTS

- Gastroesophageal reflux disease (GERD) and Barrett esophagus (BE) have been considered to be the most important risk factors for esophageal adenocarcinoma (EAC). Emerging data indicate that high-risk human papillomavirus (hr-HPV) maybe an etiologic factor for a subset of Barrett dysplasia and EAC.
- The cancer risk in BE has to be managed and involves prevention (surveillance endoscopy), treating underlying GERD, and endoscopic therapy to remove diseased epithelium in appropriate patient subgroups.
- Potential markers of dysplasia or neoplasia in BE (eg, overexpression and hr-HPV) provide an opportunity to classify patients into high and low risk groups in relation to advancing to dysplasia and EAC and thus more intensive surveillance and targeted treatment.

INTRODUCTION

Advanced esophageal adenocarcinoma (EAC) has a poor prognosis with a 5-year survival rate of less than 15%.[1,2] Conversely, patients with early-stage esophageal malignancy (stage of tumor [T]-1) (representing <10% of those undergoing esophagectomy) have a more than 90% survival rate at 5 years.[3] Gastroesophageal reflux disease (GERD) and Barrett esophagus (BE) are the most important known risk factors (as yet) for esophageal adenocarcinoma. In a study by Lagergren and colleagues,[4] persons

[a] Sam Fayad Gastro-Intestinal Viral Oncology Group, Ingham Institute for Applied Medical Research, South Western Sydney Clinical School, University of New South Wales, Liverpool, Sydney, New South Wales 2170, Australia; [b] Department of Gastroenterology & Hepatology, Bankstown-Lidcombe Hospital, South Western Sydney Local Health Network, 68-70, Eldridge Road, Bankstown, Sydney, New South Wales 2200, Australia; [c] Division of Gastroenterology and Hepatology, Veterans Affairs Medical Center, University of Kansas School of Medicine, 3901 Rainbow Boulevard, Kansas City, MO 66160, USA
* Corresponding author. Department of Gastroenterology & Hepatology, Bankstown-Lidcombe Hospital, South Western Sydney Local Health Network, 68-70, Eldridge Road, Bankstown, Sydney, New South Wales 2200, Australia.
E-mail address: Shan.Rajendra@sswahs.nsw.gov.au

Hematol Oncol Clin N Am 31 (2017) 409–426
http://dx.doi.org/10.1016/j.hoc.2017.01.003
hemonc.theclinics.com
0889-8588/17/Crown Copyright © 2017 Published by Elsevier Inc. All rights reserved.

with chronic frequent and severe GERD symptoms had an odds ratio (OR) of 43.5 for EAC. Currently, BE is the only recognized visible precursor lesion for EAC with a malignant potential currently estimated at between 0.1% and 0.3% per annum.[5,6] Esophageal cancers arising without an appreciable precursor lesion is a distinct possibility.[7] BE is defined in most countries, including the United States, as displacement of the squamocolumnar junction proximal to the gastroesophageal junction (GEJ) with specialized intestinal metaplasia on biopsy.[8] The British Society of Gastroenterology definition differs in that it is an endoscopically apparent area above the esophagogastric junction that is suggestive of BE (salmon-colored mucosa), which is supported by the finding of columnar lined esophagus on histology (**Fig. 1**).[9] This definition negates sampling errors at index endoscopy, which may miss areas of intestinal metaplasia and thus preclude patients from entering endoscopic surveillance programs. There is a lower risk of malignant progression in patients without intestinal metaplasia (0.07% per year) compared with those with intestinal metaplasia (0.38% per year) on index biopsy.[5]

Other significant risk factors for EAC include central adiposity or BMI greater than 30,[10] smoking,[11] and family history of BE or EAC.[12,13] More recently, high-risk (hr) human papillomavirus HPV (HPV) has been incriminated in a subset of patients with BE dysplasia and EAC (**Figs. 2** and **3**).[14–16] Importantly, distinct genomic differences have been found between HPV-positive and HPV-negative EACs. HPV-positive malignancies have approximately 50% less nonsilent mutations compared with virus-negative esophageal cancer. TP53 aberrations were absent in the HPV-positive EAC group, whereas 50% of the HPV-negative patients with EAC exhibited TP53 mutations. These data indicate different biological mechanisms of tumor formation.[17] An earlier study found that Barrett dysplasia (BD) and intramucosal EAC samples positive for transcriptional markers of HPV activity were mostly devoid of p53 overexpression (>80%).[16] Next-generation nucleotide sequencing revealed that almost all biologically active hr-HPV patients had detectable wildtype TP53, a hallmark of HPV-driven cancers, as is the case with cervical and head and neck malignancies.[16,18] Together, the data suggest at least 2 different carcinogenic pathways operating in EAC as has been demonstrated in head and neck tumors.[7,16,17,19,20]

Surveillance studies have demonstrated that esophageal cancer develops through a multistep pathway, the so-called Barrett metaplasia-dysplasia-adenocarcinoma

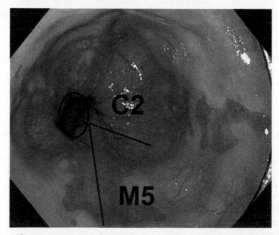

Fig. 1. Prague classification: circumference (C) and maximum (M) extent. Patient with 5 cm-long Barrett, distal 2-cm circumferential, and proximal 3 cm in form of a tongue. Barrett: C2M5.

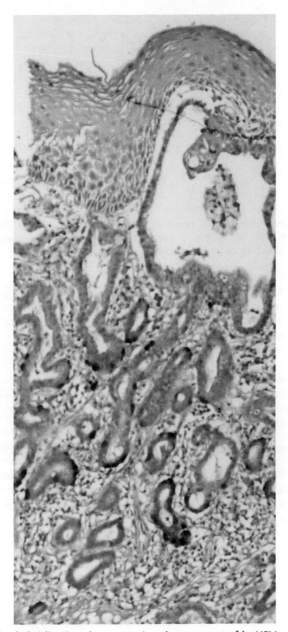

Fig. 2. DNA in situ hybridization demonstrating the presence of hr-HPV genome in esophageal adenocarcinoma tissue.

sequence.[21] Despite endoscopic surveillance, the incidence of EAC has increased almost 6-fold in the United States between 1975 and 2001 (from 4 to 23 cases per million) and is thought to represent a real increase in burden rather than a result of histologic or anatomic misclassification or overdiagnosis.[22] Recently, the rate of increase has diminished and plateaued in the United States and Sweden.[23,24] This epidemic of EAC has occurred against a backdrop of progressive reduction in the risk estimate of

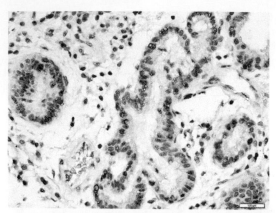

Fig. 3. RNA in situ hybridization revealing the presence of hr-HPV 16 and 18 E6/E7 messenger RNA (mRNA) in EAC tissue. Positive staining is diffusely present in the nuclei and cytoplasm as punctate or granular appearance.

malignancy associated with BE, throwing open the possibility of other causes, such as hr-HPV.[25] It has been postulated that the exponential increase in EAC is due to increasing prevalence of GERD as a result of increasing abdominal adiposity (but the rate of increase has been greater than other cancers associated with obesity), reduced prevalence rates of *Helicobacter pylori* infection, and increased ingestion of refined food with a concomitant reduction in consumption of fruit and vegetables.[25,26] It is possible that hr-HPV may be among the missing strong risk factors responsible for the significant increase of this malignancy since the 1970s. It parallels the dramatic 350% increase in head and neck squamous cell carcinoma (a well-recognized HPV-driven cancer) in the same time frame.[27–29]

EPIDEMIOLOGY, GENETICS, AND NATURAL HISTORY OF BARRETT ESOPHAGUS

BE affects predominantly white[30] and South Asian[31] men,[32] and is associated with age older than 50 years,[5] chronic GERD,[30,33] hiatal hernia,[34] and abdominal adiposity.[35] This premalignant lesion is estimated to affect between 1.6% of the adult Swedish population[36] and 6.8% of Americans.[37] Ethnic differences in the prevalence of heartburn, esophagitis, and BE are well-documented.[31,38,39] These racial differences; familial aggregation of GERD symptoms, BE, or adenocarcinoma; and twin studies suggest the possibility of a genetic component to GERD and BE.[40] A study of GERD symptoms in 8411 Swedish twin pairs older than age 55 years found a casewise concordance for GERD of 31% among female monozygotic (MZ) twins compared with 21% in female dizygotic (DZ) twins.[41]

Heritability was estimated to account for 30% of the liability to GERD. A British study of 1960 twin pairs to determine the relative contribution of genetic and environmental influences revealed that casewise concordance was significantly higher for MZ than DZ twins (42% v 26%; $P<.001$).[42] Multifactorial liability threshold modeling suggested that 43% of the variation in liability to GERD was due to multiple small genetic effects.

Genome-wide association studies have found an association between BE and 2 variants on chromosome 6p21 (major histocompatibility complex [MHC]) and 16q24 compared with controls.[43] The association of these variants with EAC was validated in another case-control study.[44] Interestingly, in a small prospective study involving multiethnic South East Asian subjects, a strong association between

HLA-B7 (0702/0706) (MHC class I) and BE in Indians (who have a white genetic make-up) compared with South Asian controls has been demonstrated.[45] Furthermore, loss of MHC class I and gain of class II were observed to be early events in BE.[46] Environmental factors (eg, *H pylori* infection) may be protective for BE in both Asians and whites.[47,48]

In those patients with chronic GERD, the prevalence of BE is 10% to 15%.[49] A large proportion of patients with BE are asymptomatic and almost all (>90%) never progress to EAC.[50] Two large population-based studies have determined the risk estimate of cancer in nondysplastic BE (NDBE) to be between 0.12% and 0.13%.[5,6]

The malignancy potential in Barrett low-grade dysplasia (LGD) is poorly defined[13] due to poor interobserver correlation, biopsy sampling error, and regression of LGD as a result of immunosurveillance.[51–54] The incidence of EAC among patients with Barrett LGD is estimated at between 0.5% and 0.6% per year.[6,54,55] In a meta-analysis involving 4 studies that included subjects with high-grade dysplasia (HGD) but excluded prevalent cancers and those subjects with previous endoscopic and/or surgical intervention, the incidence of EAC was estimated to be between 5.6% and 6.6% per annum.[56]

PREDICTORS OF PROGRESSION (ENDOSCOPIC, HISTOLOGIC, AND MOLECULAR)

The longer the segment of BE, the greater the risk of progression to HGD or EAC.[57,58] A multicenter study that enrolled 1175 subjects with NDBE with a mean follow-up of 5.5 years revealed that BE length predicted the risk of progression to HGD or EAC with an OR of 1.2. Every 1 cm increase in length resulted in a 28% greater risk for neoplasia.[59]

Currently, dysplasia is considered the best (but imprecise) marker of cancer risk in BE. Given the shortcomings of dysplasia as a cancer risk stratification tool, especially in low-grade, as mentioned previously, several biomarkers have been proposed to predict the risk of malignant progression.

P53 immunohistochemistry has been proposed as a good clinical molecular marker for predicting disease progression in BD[60,61] and, as such, has been recommended as an adjunct to routine clinical diagnosis by the British Society of Gastroenterology.[12] Nevertheless, there is wide variability in positive staining for overexpression, in the order of between 50% and 90%.[62,63] TP53 mutations due to frame-shifts, deletions, defective splice sites, or nonsense mutations can all result in absent p53 staining.[64] HPV E6 oncoprotein-mediated degradation of TP53 is another cause of negative staining for p53 in BD or EAC.[16,17,65] A recent discovery that hr-HPV is strongly associated with a subset of patients with BD and EAC should prompt further investigation in the use of biomarkers relating to viral transcriptional activity (p16INK4A, E6/E7mRNA) to identify the high-risk group of progressors to malignancy.[14–16]

Chromosome instability (the most common cause of genomic instability) is strongly associated with progression from BE to EAC.[66] A study involving 243 subjects with BE in whom esophageal biopsies were subjected to a chromosome instability biomarker panel consisting of 9p loss of heterozygosity (LOH) (inactivation of p16), 17p LOH (inactivation of p53), and aneuploidy or tetraploidy (DNA content abnormalities) revealed that those who tested positive for all of the above had a relative risk of progression to EAC of 38.7 (95% CI 10.8–138.5).[67] Genetic clonal diversity in BE has been shown to predict progression to EAC even after controlling for genetic factors (eg TP53 and ploidy abnormalities). Specifically, 3 clones double the risk of progression to cancer.[68] An increase in copy number and its variation,[69] as well as catastrophic genomic events, have been shown to precede carcinogenesis in up to 32% of EAC cases.[70]

Using a text-mining methodology, Kalatskaya[71] determined that TP53 (p53), CDKN2A (p16INK4A), CTNNB1 (β-catenin), CDH1 (E-cadherin), GPX3 (glutathione peroxidase 3), and NOX5 (NADPH oxidase 5) were the top candidate genes involved in BE progression to cancer. These 6 functionally interrelated genes are involved in a diverse range of biological pathways, including DNA repair (TP53), cell cycle (TP53, CDKN2A), regulation of cell-cell adhesion or gene transcription (CTNNB1), cellular adhesion (CDH1), and detoxification of reactive oxygen species (GPX3, NOX5), and are subject to genomic, transcriptomic, and proteomic alterations in a significant proportion of EACs.[71]

SCREENING FOR BARRETT ESOPHAGUS

Patients at risk of EAC (ie, age 50 years or older, white, male, chronic GERD, hiatal hernia, abdominal adiposity and elevated body mass index, and family history of EAC) should be screened with either standard esophagogastroduodenoscopy or transnasal endoscopy.[13,72,73] Nevertheless, there are no prospective, randomized, controlled trials demonstrating benefit in terms of decreasing the incidence or mortality of EAC or cost-effectiveness in screening for BE. Screening the general population with GERD for BE is not currently recommended and individualized screening has been suggested because reflux symptoms are not a reliable marker for BE.[13,36,37]

ENDOSCOPIC SURVEILLANCE OF BARRETT ESOPHAGUS

Current management strategy is to enroll patients with BE into surveillance programs in an attempt to detect cancer at an early and potentially curable stage. The current recommendations for surveillance in BE are to perform endoscopy every 3 to 5 years.[8,13] Patients with LGD who undergo endoscopic surveillance should do so at intervals of 6 to 12 months and those with HGD in the absence of eradication therapy should do so every 3 months. The American Gastroenterological Association (AGA) recommends endoscopic eradication therapy rather than surveillance for treatment of patients with HGD.[13] The finding of dysplasia needs to be confirmed by an independent second pathologist to reduce interobserver variation. Patients with dysplasia should be on proton pump inhibitor (PPI) therapy to reduce inflammatory changes that could make histopathological interpretation difficult.

BARRETT ESOPHAGUS EVALUATION

Assessment for BE is done if the squamocolumnar junction is located above the GEJ. BE is measured from the proximal (top) end of the longitudinal gastric folds at the GEJ to the area of columnar epithelium that terminates at the site of the squamocolumnar demarcation. BE has been traditionally defined as long segment (>3 cm) and short segment (≤3 cm). The Prague criteria have superseded it and identify the circumferential (C) and maximum (M) extent of Barrett metaplasia (see **Fig. 1**). It has been demonstrated to have excellent interobserver agreement among endoscopists (for columnar epithelium extending at least 1 cm above the GEJ).[74] Endoscopic evaluation of the columnar-lined esophagus is carefully performed using high-resolution white light endoscopy or electronic or dye chromoendoscopy.[13] Four quadrant biopsy specimens are obtained every 1 to 2 cm, as well as targeted biopsies of apparent lesions from patients with BE.[74,75] In patients with known or suspected BD, 4 quadrant biopsy specimens are obtained every 1 cm.[13] Specific biopsy specimens of any mucosal irregularity are sent separately to the pathologist for evaluation.[50,74]

It is recommended that endoscopists who evaluate patients for BE using high-definition white light endoscopy spend an average of 1 minute per centimeter of BE before obtaining biopsies.[76] It is unclear if inspection time is directly responsible for improved detection rates or a surrogate marker for more obsessive and observant endoscopists.

MANAGEMENT OBJECTIVES IN BARRETT ESOPHAGUS

The 3 main objectives in managing BE are treating GERD (medically and or surgically), cancer prevention (including the previously mentioned surveillance), and endoscopic therapy to remove diseased epithelium in appropriate patient subgroups.

MANAGEMENT OF UNDERLYING GASTROESOPHAGEAL REFLUX DISEASE

- Life-style modification: weight loss, eating small frequent meals, avoiding acidic and spicy foods, and raising the head of the bed by 6 inches.[77,78]
- PPIs are the mainstay of treatment.
- H2-receptor antagonists may be required to combat nocturnal acid breakthrough.
- Prokinetic therapy may help volume regurgitation. Domperidone is unavailable in the United States but metoclopramide is a suitable alternative. The use of cisapride has been severely restricted worldwide given its propensity to cause a fatal form of ventricular arrhythmia (torsades de pointes) in the presence of QT prolongation.
- Baclofen, a gamma-aminobutyric acid-B (GABA $_B$) receptor agonist reduces transient lower esophageal sphincter relaxations and may be effective in patients with upright reflux and belching.[79] Its side-effect profile of drowsiness, dizziness, nausea or vomiting, seizures, and potential death on withdrawal has precluded its widespread use for refractory GERD.
- Almost all studies involving medical therapy for BE use either resolution of reflux symptoms or normalization of esophageal acid exposure as the endpoint.[25] The former is a poor predictor of persistent acid reflux in patients with BE[80] and there are insufficient data advocating esophageal pH monitoring to optimize PPI therapy to fully control reflux symptoms.
- An antireflux operation can be considered, most commonly a Nissen fundoplication, in patients with significant volume regurgitation or those responding to medical therapy but wanting a surgical alternative. This involves wrapping a portion of the gastric fundus around the distal esophagus and closing the crura (to prevent the esophagus sliding out). Surgical intervention should be preceded by pH-metry (to confirm pathologic reflux) and manometry (to exclude underlying esophageal motility problems). Early complications include pneumothorax, surgical emphysema, perforation, and transient dysphagia. Late postoperative complications are gas-bloat syndrome, dysphagia, and small bowel obstruction.
- It is worth noting that neither surgery nor medical therapy have been shown to prevent EAC.[13]

CHEMOPREVENTION IN BARRETT ESOPHAGUS

Indirect evidence exists to support the use of PPIs as a chemopreventive agent in BE. In a randomized control trial involving BE subjects treated with PPI versus histamine type II receptor blockers, there was an 8% regression in BE surface area in the former group.[81] An inverse correlation has been established between long-term use of PPIs and the incidence of dysplasia and adenocarcinoma in BE.[82–84] Nevertheless, there are no prospective clinical studies demonstrating that PPI therapy prevents the development of dysplasia and progression to cancer.

Nonsteroidal Anti-inflammatory Drugs

A meta-analysis of 9 clinical studies has shown a 43% decreased rate of esophageal cancer in subjects who use nonsteroidal anti-inflammatory drugs (NSAIDs).[85] A 50% reduction of esophageal malignancy was seen with aspirin use. In a prospective study involving 350 subjects with BE followed up for a median of 65.5 months, there was a reduced risk of EAC in current users of NSAIDs (hazard ratio 0.20, 95% CI 0.10–0.41) versus subjects who had never used these drugs.[86] Inhibition of cyclooxygenase-2 and immunomodulation by NSAIDs has been postulated as the mechanism for the prevention of progression of BE to adenocarcinoma.[87,88] A negative study involving a cyclooxygenase-2 selective NSAID and BE was reported by Heath and colleagues.[89] The Aspirin Esomeprazole Chemoprevention Trial (ASPECT) in BE is currently investigating if treating with aspirin and high-dose PPIs can reduce progression from metaplasia-dysplasia-adenocarcinoma and hence reduce mortality. In the interim, it is appropriate to consider prescription of low-dose aspirin for BE subjects (who are already on a PPI) with concomitant risk factors for cardiovascular disease.[13]

Statin use is associated with a lower risk of cancer in patients with BE. A meta-analysis revealed a 41% reduction in the risk of EAC in 2125 subjects with BE (number needed to treat = 389).[90] In a recently published nested case (EAC, n = 311) control (n = 856) study, statin use was inversely associated with development of EAC (OR 0.65, 95% CI 0.47–0.91).[91]

ERADICATION OF DYSPLASIA AND REDUCTION OF PROGRESSION TO ESOPHAGEAL ADENOCARCINOMA

Complete eradication of dysplasia and hence reduction of progression to esophageal adenocarcinoma can be achieved by endoscopic means or via surgery (**Fig. 4**). Elimination of metaplastic or dysplastic cells involves ablation, endoscopic mucosal resection (EMR) and esophagectomy. Ablation can take the form of heat injury (multipolar electrocautery, argon plasma coagulation, laser, neodymium-doped yttrium aluminum garnet, radiofrequency ablation [RFA], cryotherapy, and photochemical injury).

Current interest is mainly focused on RFA, which is a relatively new endoscopic treatment modality for BE or intramucosal adenocarcinoma consisting of a balloon-based bipolar radiofrequency ablation catheter (balloon or probe), sizing catheters, and a radiofrequency energy generator. This mode of endoscopic eradication therapy is favored by most endoscopists for flat lesions, whereas EMR is suitable for raised or nodular lesions. Endoscopic spray cryotherapy ablation uses liquid nitrogen ($-196°C$, CSA Medical system, CSA Medical Inc, Lexington, MA) or rapidly expanding carbon dioxide gas ($-78°C$ at flow temperature of 6–8 L/min, Polar Wand GI Supply, Camp Hill, PA) to produce rapid freezing and slow thawing of a defined volume of tissue-causing injury. This technique is preferred by some endoscopists and can be useful in those patients refractory to RFA. After ablation or EMR, antisecretory therapy in the form of PPIs is prescribed, so the esophageal mucosa heals with the growth of new squamous epithelium (neosquamous epithelium).

NONDYSPLASTIC BARRETT ESOPHAGUS

The use of invasive ablative therapies in NDBE is difficult to justify given the low risk for malignancy in Barrett metaplasia[92]; the inadequately understood natural history of

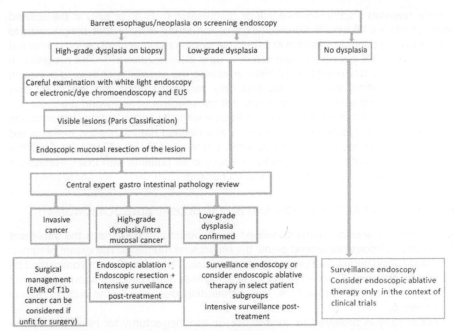

Fig. 4. Algorithm for management of BE and intramucosal adenocarcinoma. EMR, endoscopic mucosal resection; EUS, endoscopic ultrasound; T1b, tumor invades submucosa. (*Adapted from* Rajendra S, Sharma P. Management of Barrett's oesophagus and intramucosal oesophageal cancer: a review of recent development. Therap Adv Gastroenterol 2012;5(5):294; with permission.)

this condition, which has so far precluded identifying the high-risk population of progressors to EAC[25]; and the potential for complications with endotherapy. Moreover, patients with BE have the same life expectancy as does the general population.[52]

It has also been shown that RFA for NDBE was not cost-effective compared with endoscopic surveillance and ablation if HGD develops.[93]

Thus, currently, endoscopic surveillance for NDBE is recommended by most gastroenterology societies worldwide. Nevertheless, there are no data to back this practice in relation to reducing mortality from EAC.[7,94]

Standard surveillance protocol in the UK and United States recommends 2 to 5 yearly surveillance endoscopies.[8,12,13] Four quadrant biopsy specimens should be obtained every 1 to 2 cm, as well as targeted biopsies of apparent lesions from patients with BE. The recent guidelines from the UK have advocated endoscopic surveillance only in BE patients with biopsies showing intestinal metaplasia; individuals with short-segment BE, 3 to 5 yearly; and those with long-segment BE, 2 to 3 yearly.[12]

BARRETT LOW-GRADE DYSPLASIA

Dysplasia must be confirmed by at least 2 expert gastrointestinal (GI) pathologists before contemplating 1 of 2 options: surveillance or eradication of the diseased mucosa.[13]

If surveillance is undertaken, the next endoscopy should be within 6 months after the index examination with a diagnosis of LGD. If no progression of dysplasia is detected, annual endoscopy until no dysplasia for 2 consecutive years, after which the nondysplastic surveillance protocol could be adopted.

A more recent prospective randomized controlled trial of subjects with LGD treated with RFA (n = 68) or subjected to endoscopic surveillance (n = 68) and followed up for

3 years revealed a 25% reduced risk of progression to HGD or EAC in the ablated group (1.5% vs 26.5%).[95] Shortcomings of the study include that progression to HGD or EAC in controls was high at 11.8% per person per year of follow-up compared with 1.4% to 1.8% per person year of follow-up in other studies.[5,6,51] This progression occurred mainly within the first 12 months, raising the possibility of missed prevalent lesions. In addition, the diagnosis was only confirmed once and the study only involved expert referral centers that may not be reflective of real-world practice.

Given that the definition of dysplasia is fraught with difficulties (notably inflammation masquerading as dysplasia) and without a well-defined natural history, exacerbated by widely varying risk estimates for progression to cancer of 0.6% to 1.6%,[74,96–99] it is difficult to be definite about ablative therapy in all patients with LGD. Perhaps, it could be considered in a subgroup of LGD patients.

BARRETT HIGH-GRADE DYSPLASIA AND INTRAMUCOSAL ADENOCARCINOMA

Intramucosal adenocarcinoma is defined as neoplasia that penetrates the basement membrane but does not extend below the muscularis mucosae. The extent of tumor, spread to lymph nodes, and presence of metastasis (TNM classification) developed by the American Joint Committee on Cancer defines intramucosal adenocarcinoma confined to the mucosa as T1m, that penetrating deeper into the submucosa as T1sm (**Fig. 5**).

Endotherapy is preferred to surveillance or esophagectomy for HGD or intramucosal cancer but all such patients should be discussed at the multidisciplinary meeting involving the GI pathologist (preferably with an interest in esophageal diseases), interventional endoscopist, upper-GI surgeon, and medical oncologist or radiotherapist.

The combination of EMR and ablative therapy, particularly RFA, has replaced esophagectomy as the standard of care in the management of HGD and esophageal intramucosal cancer (that has not breached the muscularis mucosae). Endoscopic ablative therapy should be undertaken in centers of excellence where ablative skills, patient volume, and specialized care are optimal.

Endoscopic ultrasound using the TNM classification is useful in deciding whether patients with adenocarcinoma are offered endoscopic therapy or esophagectomy.[25]

Before EMR is performed, gross tumor morphology is assessed using the Paris classification (type I, protruding; type II a, slightly elevated; type II b, completely flat; type II c, slightly depressed; type III, excavated).

All visible (nodular) lesions should undergo EMR (histologic assessment of the whole lesion permitting definition of lateral extent plus depth). Complications of EMR include stricture formation, hemorrhage, and perforation.

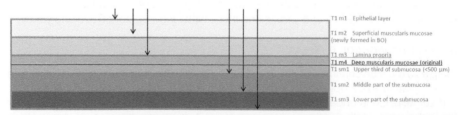

Fig. 5. Intramucosal Barrett adenocarcinoma (T1) subclassification. Lymph node metastases in intramucosal cancer are 1% to 2% and that involving the upper third of the submucosa is between 0% and 8%. (*Adapted from* Rajendra S, Sharma P. Management of Barrett's oesophagus and intramucosal oesophageal cancer: a review of recent development. Therap Adv Gastroenterol 2012;5(5):291; with permission.)

Mucosally confined esophageal carcinoma has a very low risk of metastatic lymphadenopathy (1%–2%), which makes endoscopic resection feasible.[100]

RFA is currently the ablative therapy of choice for flat dysplastic or neoplastic epithelium. In the Ablation of Intestinal Metaplasia containing Dysplasia trial (AIM dysplasia) (HGD = 63), complete eradication of HGD occurred in 81% of those in the ablation group compared with 19% in the control group. In the HGD group, complete eradication of dysplasia was achieved in 95% at 2 years and 96% at 3 years.[101,102]

Nonrandomized and uncontrolled studies show success rates for cryotherapy comparable to RFA for the treatment of Barrett HGD, with complete eradication of dysplasia seen in 87% to 96%, and complete elimination of intestinal metaplasia in 57% to 96%, of treated patients.[103–105] In early-stage esophageal cancer, spray cryotherapy eliminates mucosal cancer in 75% of patients.[105]

All patients should be on high-dose PPI therapy twice daily during and after treatment and continue to have lifelong endoscopic surveillance.

If the neoplasia has breached the muscularis mucosae, the submucosa is then, by definition, involved and lymph node metastases are in the order of 10% to 20% and esophagectomy (distal or subtotal) is indicated.[106] Nevertheless, some investigators have reported that the upper third of the submucosa (sm1) has a very low risk of lymph node metastasis.[107,108] Others have reported a risk of lymph node involvement of between 0% and 8% and even as high as 12.9% in sm1 esophageal adenocarcinoma.[109–111] Thus, the jury is still out as to whether sm1 cancers might be eligible for endoscopic resection with a curative intent.

Historically, the gold standard for treatment of HGD and intramucosal cancer was esophagectomy.

The 5-year survival rate in patients postesophagectomy is between 90% and 95%. Significant morbidity occurs in approximately 40% to 50%, including pulmonary complications, anastomotic leak, dysphagia, loss of appetite, early satiety, fatigue, and loss of functional esophagus.[112–114] Esophagectomies should be performed by an experienced surgeon in a high-volume center to minimize morbidity and mortality (4.9% at a center performing >50 esophagectomies).[115]

SUMMARY

Despite screening, surveillance, new developments in imaging and molecular markers, as well as the armamentarium of ablative therapy available to the endoscopist, there has been no reduction in EAC in the Western world. Future research must be focused on fine-tuning the screening and surveillance programs to identify more accurately the high-risk group of progressors to EAC who would benefit most from ablative therapy. The availability of potential markers of dysplasia or neoplasia in BE (ie, p53 immunohistochemistry or nucleotide sequencing and hr-HPV) provides an opportunity to classify patients into high-risk and low-risk groups in relation to advancing to dysplasia and EAC and thus to more intensive surveillance.[7] In the very near future, genome-wide technology may provide molecular signatures to further refine diagnosis and risk stratification in BE.

REFERENCES

1. Pondugula K, Wani S, Sharma P. Barrett's esophagus and esophageal adenocarcinoma in adults: long-term GERD or something else? Curr Gastroenterol Rep 2007;9:468–74.
2. Eloubeidi MA, Provenzale D. Health-related quality of life and severity of symptoms in patients with Barrett's esophagus and gastroesophageal reflux disease patients without Barrett's esophagus. Am J Gastroenterol 2000;95:1881–7.

3. Visbal AL, Allen MS, Miller DL, et al. Ivor Lewis esophagogastrectomy for esophageal cancer. Ann Thorac Surg 2001;71:1803–8.
4. Lagergren J, Bergstrom R, Lindgren A, et al. Symptomatic gastroesophageal reflux as a risk factor for esophageal adenocarcinoma. N Engl J Med 1999; 340:825–31.
5. Bhat S, Coleman HG, Yousef F, et al. Risk of malignant progression in Barrett's esophagus patients: results from a large population-based study. J Natl Cancer Inst 2011;103:1049–57.
6. Hvid-Jensen F, Pedersen L, Drewes AM, et al. Incidence of adenocarcinoma among patients with Barrett's esophagus. N Engl J Med 2011;365:1375–83.
7. Rajendra S. Barrett's oesophagus: can meaningful screening and surveillance guidelines be formulated based on new data and rejigging the old paradigm? Best Pract Res Clin Gastroenterol 2015;29:65–75.
8. Wang KK, Sampliner RE, Practice Parameters Committee of the American College of Gastroenterology. Updated guidelines 2008 for the diagnosis, surveillance and therapy of Barrett's esophagus. Am J Gastroenterol 2008;103: 788–97.
9. Playford RJ. New British Society of Gastroenterology (BSG) guidelines for the diagnosis and management of Barrett's oesophagus. Gut 2006;55:442.
10. Turati F, Tramacere I, La Vecchia C, et al. A meta-analysis of body mass index and esophageal and gastric cardia adenocarcinoma. Ann Oncol 2013;24: 609–17.
11. Coleman HG, Bhat S, Johnston BT, et al. Tobacco smoking increases the risk of high-grade dysplasia and cancer among patients with Barrett's esophagus. Gastroenterology 2012;142:233–40.
12. Fitzgerald RC, di Pietro M, Ragunath K, et al. British Society of Gastroenterology guidelines on the diagnosis and management of Barrett's oesophagus. Gut 2014;63:7–42.
13. Spechler SJ, Sharma P, Souza RF, et al. American Gastroenterological Association technical review on the management of Barrett's esophagus. Gastroenterology 2011;140:e18–52 [quiz: e13].
14. Rajendra S, Wang B, Snow ET, et al. Transcriptionally active human papillomavirus is strongly associated with Barrett's dysplasia and esophageal adenocarcinoma. Am J Gastroenterol 2013;108:1082–93.
15. Wang B, Rajendra S, Pavey D, et al. Viral load and integration status of high-risk human papillomaviruses in the Barrett's metaplasia-dysplasia-adenocarcinoma sequence. Am J Gastroenterol 2013;108:1814–6.
16. Rajendra S, Wang B, Pavey D, et al. Persistence of human papillomavirus, overexpression of p53, and outcomes of patients after endoscopic ablation of Barrett's esophagus. Clin Gastroenterol Hepatol 2015;13:1364–8.e5.
17. Rajendra S, Wang B, Merrett N, et al. Genomic analysis of HPV-positive versus HPV-negative oesophageal adenocarcinoma identifies a differential mutational landscape. J Med Genet 2016;53:227–31.
18. Ojesina AI, Lichtenstein L, Freeman SS, et al. Landscape of genomic alterations in cervical carcinomas. Nature 2014;506:371–5.
19. Brennan JA, Boyle JO, Koch WM, et al. Association between cigarette smoking and mutation of the p53 gene in squamous-cell carcinoma of the head and neck. N Engl J Med 1995;332:712–7.
20. Gillison ML, Koch WM, Capone RB, et al. Evidence for a causal association between human papillomavirus and a subset of head and neck cancers. J Natl Cancer Inst 2000;92:709–20.

21. Jankowski JA, Wright NA, Meltzer SJ, et al. Molecular evolution of the metaplasia-dysplasia-adenocarcinoma sequence in the esophagus. Am J Pathol 1999;154:965–73.

22. Pohl H, Welch HG. The role of overdiagnosis and reclassification in the marked increase of esophageal adenocarcinoma incidence. J Natl Cancer Inst 2005;97: 142–6.

23. Pohl H, Sirovich B, Welch HG. Esophageal adenocarcinoma incidence: are we reaching the peak? Cancer Epidemiol Biomarkers Prev 2010;19:1468–70.

24. Lagergren J, Mattsson F. No further increase in the incidence of esophageal adenocarcinoma in Sweden. Int J Cancer 2011;129:513–6.

25. Rajendra S, Sharma P. Management of Barrett's oesophagus and intramucosal oesophageal cancer: a review of recent development. Therap Adv Gastroenterol 2012;5:285–99.

26. Buas MF, Vaughan TL. Epidemiology and risk factors for gastroesophageal junction tumors: understanding the rising incidence of this disease. Semin Radiat Oncol 2013;23:3–9.

27. Chaturvedi AK, Engels EA, Pfeiffer RM, et al. Human papillomavirus and rising oropharyngeal cancer incidence in the United States. J Clin Oncol 2011;29: 4294–301.

28. Nasman A, Attner P, Hammarstedt L, et al. Incidence of human papillomavirus (HPV) positive tonsillar carcinoma in Stockholm, Sweden: an epidemic of viral-induced carcinoma? Int J Cancer 2009;125:362–6.

29. Hocking JS, Stein A, Conway EL, et al. Head and neck cancer in Australia between 1982 and 2005 show increasing incidence of potentially HPV-associated oropharyngeal cancers. Br J Cancer 2011;104:886–91.

30. Corley DA, Kubo A, Levin TR, et al. Race, ethnicity, sex and temporal differences in Barrett's oesophagus diagnosis: a large community-based study, 1994-2006. Gut 2009;58:182–8.

31. Rajendra S, Kutty K, Karim N. Ethnic differences in the prevalence of endoscopic esophagitis and Barrett's esophagus: the long and short of it all. Dig Dis Sci 2004;49:237–42.

32. Cook MB, Chow WH, Devesa SS. Oesophageal cancer incidence in the United States by race, sex, and histologic type, 1977-2005. Br J Cancer 2009;101: 855–9.

33. Edelstein ZR, Bronner MP, Rosen SN, et al. Risk factors for Barrett's esophagus among patients with gastroesophageal reflux disease: a community clinic-based case-control study. Am J Gastroenterol 2009;104:834–42.

34. Westhoff B, Brotze S, Weston A, et al. The frequency of Barrett's esophagus in high-risk patients with chronic GERD. Gastrointest Endosc 2005;61:226–31.

35. Edelstein ZR, Farrow DC, Bronner MP, et al. Central adiposity and risk of Barrett's esophagus. Gastroenterology 2007;133:403–11.

36. Ronkainen J, Aro P, Storskrubb T, et al. High prevalence of gastroesophageal reflux symptoms and esophagitis with or without symptoms in the general adult Swedish population: a Kalixanda study report. Scand J Gastroenterol 2005;40: 275–85.

37. Rex DK, Cummings OW, Shaw M, et al. Screening for Barrett's esophagus in colonoscopy patients with and without heartburn. Gastroenterology 2003;125: 1670–7.

38. Rajendra S, Alahuddin S. Racial differences in the prevalence of heartburn. Aliment Pharmacol Ther 2004;19:375–6.

39. Cameron A. Molecular biology of Barrett's esophagus. In: Sharma P, Sampliner R, editors. Barrett's Esophagus and esophageal adenocarcinoma. Malden (MA): Blackwell Publishing; 2006. p. 82–91.

40. Chak A, Lee T, Kinnard MF, et al. Familial aggregation of Barrett's oesophagus, oesophageal adenocarcinoma, and oesophagogastric junctional adenocarcinoma in Caucasian adults. Gut 2002;51:323–8.

41. Cameron AJ, Lagergren J, Henriksson C, et al. Gastroesophageal reflux disease in monozygotic and dizygotic twins. Gastroenterology 2002;122:55–9.

42. Mohammed I, Cherkas LF, Riley SA, et al. Genetic influences in gastro-oesophageal reflux disease: a twin study. Gut 2003;52:1085–9.

43. Su Z, Gay LJ, Strange A, et al. Common variants at the MHC locus and at chromosome 16q24.1 predispose to Barrett's esophagus. Nat Genet 2012;44: 1131–6.

44. Dura P, van Veen EM, Salomon J, et al. Barrett associated MHC and FOXF1 variants also increase esophageal carcinoma risk. Int J Cancer 2013;133:1751–5.

45. Rajendra S, Ackroyd R, Murad S, et al. Human leucocyte antigen determinants of susceptibility to Barrett's oesophagus in Asians–a preliminary study. Aliment Pharmacol Ther 2005;21:1377–83.

46. Rajendra S, Ackroyd R, Karim N, et al. Loss of human leucocyte antigen class I and gain of class II expression are early events in carcinogenesis: clues from a study of Barrett's oesophagus. J Clin Pathol 2006;59:952–7.

47. Rajendra S, Ackroyd R, Robertson IK, et al. Helicobacter pylori, ethnicity, and the gastroesophageal reflux disease spectrum: a study from the East. Helicobacter 2007;12:177–83.

48. Corley DA, Kubo A, Levin TR, et al. Helicobacter pylori infection and the risk of Barrett's oesophagus: a community-based study. Gut 2008;57:727–33.

49. Sharma P. Clinical practice. Barrett's esophagus. N Engl J Med 2009;361: 2548–56.

50. Reid BJ, Blount PL, Feng Z, et al. Optimizing endoscopic biopsy detection of early cancers in Barrett's high-grade dysplasia. Am J Gastroenterol 2000;95: 3089–96.

51. Wani S, Falk GW, Post J, et al. Risk factors for progression of low-grade dysplasia in patients with Barrett's esophagus. Gastroenterology 2011;141: 1179–86, 1186.e1.

52. Sharma P, McQuaid K, Dent J, et al. A critical review of the diagnosis and management of Barrett's esophagus: the AGA Chicago Workshop. Gastroenterology 2004;127:310–30.

53. Rajendra S, Robertson IK. Similar immunogenetics of Barrett's oesophagus and cervical neoplasia: is HPV the common denominator? J Clin Pathol 2010;63:1–3.

54. Sharma P, Falk GW, Weston AP, et al. Dysplasia and cancer in a large multicenter cohort of patients with Barrett's esophagus. Clin Gastroenterol Hepatol 2006;4:566–72.

55. Singh S, Manickam P, Amin AV, et al. Incidence of esophageal adenocarcinoma in Barrett's esophagus with low-grade dysplasia: a systematic review and meta-analysis. Gastrointest Endosc 2014;79:897–909.e4 [quiz: 983.e1–3].

56. Rastogi A, Puli S, El-Serag HB, et al. Incidence of esophageal adenocarcinoma in patients with Barrett's esophagus and high-grade dysplasia: a meta-analysis. Gastrointest Endosc 2008;67:394–8.

57. Weston AP, Badr AS, Hassanein RS. Prospective multivariate analysis of clinical, endoscopic, and histological factors predictive of the development of Barrett's

multifocal high-grade dysplasia or adenocarcinoma. Am J Gastroenterol 1999; 94:3413–9.

58. Thomas T, Abrams KR, De Caestecker JS, et al. Meta analysis: cancer risk in Barrett's oesophagus. Aliment Pharmacol Ther 2007;26:1465–77.

59. Anaparthy R, Gaddam S, Kanakadandi V, et al. Association between length of Barrett's esophagus and risk of high-grade dysplasia or adenocarcinoma in patients without dysplasia. Clin Gastroenterol Hepatol 2013;11:1430–6.

60. Kastelein F, Biermann K, Steyerberg EW, et al. Aberrant p53 protein expression is associated with an increased risk of neoplastic progression in patients with Barrett's oesophagus. Gut 2013;62:1676–83.

61. Bird-Lieberman EL, Dunn JM, Coleman HG, et al. Population-based study reveals new risk-stratification biomarker panel for Barrett's esophagus. Gastroenterology 2012;143:927–35.e3.

62. Kaye PV, Haider SA, James PD, et al. Novel staining pattern of p53 in Barrett's dysplasia–the absent pattern. Histopathology 2010;57:933–5.

63. Khan S, Do KA, Kuhnert P, et al. Diagnostic value of p53 immunohistochemistry in Barrett's esophagus: an endoscopic study. Pathology 1998;30:136–40.

64. Wojnarowicz PM, Oros KK, Quinn MC, et al. The genomic landscape of TP53 and p53 annotated high grade ovarian serous carcinomas from a defined founder population associated with patient outcome. PLoS One 2012;7:e45484.

65. Scheffner M, Werness BA, Huibregtse JM, et al. The E6 oncoprotein encoded by human papillomavirus types 16 and 18 promotes the degradation of p53. Cell 1990;63:1129–36.

66. Reid BJ. Early events during neoplastic progression in Barrett's esophagus. Cancer Biomark 2010;9:307–24.

67. Galipeau PC, Li X, Blount PL, et al. NSAIDs modulate CDKN2A, TP53, and DNA content risk for progression to esophageal adenocarcinoma. PLoS Med 2007;4:e67.

68. Maley CC, Galipeau PC, Finley JC, et al. Genetic clonal diversity predicts progression to esophageal adenocarcinoma. Nat Genet 2006;38:468–73.

69. Li X, Galipeau PC, Paulson TG, et al. Temporal and spatial evolution of somatic chromosomal alterations: a case-cohort study of Barrett's esophagus. Cancer Prev Res (Phila) 2014;7:114–27.

70. Nones K, Waddell N, Wayte N, et al. Genomic catastrophes frequently arise in esophageal adenocarcinoma and drive tumorigenesis. Nat Commun 2014;5: 5224.

71. Kalatskaya I. Overview of major molecular alterations during progression from Barrett's esophagus to esophageal adenocarcinoma. Ann N Y Acad Sci 2016; 1381(1):74–91.

72. Shaheen NJ, Falk GW, Iyer PG, et al. ACG clinical guideline: diagnosis and management of Barrett's esophagus. Am J Gastroenterol 2016;111:30–50 [quiz: 51].

73. Balasubramanian G, Singh M, Gupta N, et al. Prevalence and predictors of columnar lined esophagus in gastroesophageal reflux disease (GERD) patients undergoing upper endoscopy. Am J Gastroenterol 2012;107:1655–61.

74. Sharma P, Dent J, Armstrong D, et al. The development and validation of an endoscopic grading system for Barrett's esophagus: the Prague C & M criteria. Gastroenterology 2006;131:1392–9.

75. Provenzale D, Kemp JA, Arora S, et al. A guide for surveillance of patients with Barrett's esophagus. Am J Gastroenterol 1994;89:670–80.

76. Gupta N, Gaddam S, Wani SB, et al. Longer Barrett's inspection time (BIT) is associated with a higher detection rate of high grade dysplasia (HGD) and early esophageal adenocarcinoma (EAC). Gastrointest Endosc 2012;76:531–8.

77. Garud SS, Keilin S, Cai Q, et al. Diagnosis and management of Barrett's esophagus for the endoscopist. Therap Adv Gastroenterol 2010;3:227–38.

78. Harvey RF, Gordon PC, Hadley N, et al. Effects of sleeping with the bed-head raised and of ranitidine in patients with severe peptic oesophagitis. Lancet 1987;2:1200–3.

79. Cossentino MJ, Mann K, Armbruster SP, et al. Randomised clinical trial: the effect of baclofen in patients with gastro-oesophageal reflux–a randomised prospective study. Aliment Pharmacol Ther 2012;35:1036–44.

80. Gerson LB, Boparai V, Ullah N, et al. Oesophageal and gastric pH profiles in patients with gastro-oesophageal reflux disease and Barrett's oesophagus treated with proton pump inhibitors. Aliment Pharmacol Ther 2004;20:637–43.

81. Peters FT, Ganesh S, Kuipers EJ, et al. Endoscopic regression of Barrett's oesophagus during omeprazole treatment; a randomised double blind study. Gut 1999;45:489–94.

82. El-Serag HB, Aguirre TV, Davis S, et al. Proton pump inhibitors are associated with reduced incidence of dysplasia in Barrett's esophagus. Am J Gastroenterol 2004;99:1877–83.

83. Cooper BT, Chapman W, Neumann CS, et al. Continuous treatment of Barrett's oesophagus patients with proton pump inhibitors up to 13 years: observations on regression and cancer incidence. Aliment Pharmacol Ther 2006;23:727–33.

84. Nguyen DM, El-Serag HB, Henderson L, et al. Medication usage and the risk of neoplasia in patients with Barrett's esophagus. Clin Gastroenterol Hepatol 2009; 7:1299–304.

85. Corley DA, Kerlikowske K, Verma R, et al. Protective association of aspirin/NSAIDs and esophageal cancer: a systematic review and meta-analysis. Gastroenterology 2003;124:47–56.

86. Vaughan TL, Dong LM, Blount PL, et al. Non-steroidal anti-inflammatory drugs and risk of neoplastic progression in Barrett's oesophagus: a prospective study. Lancet Oncol 2005;6:945–52.

87. Jankowski J, deCaestecker J, Harrison R, et al. NSAID and oesophageal adenocarcinoma: randomised trials needed to correct for bias. Lancet Oncol 2006;7: 7–8 [author reply: 8–9].

88. Rajendra S. Immunomodulatory effects of non-steroidal anti-inflammatory drugs in Barrett's oesophagus. Lancet Oncol 2006;7:103–4.

89. Heath EI, Canto MI, Piantadosi S, et al. Secondary chemoprevention of Barrett's esophagus with celecoxib: results of a randomized trial. J Natl Cancer Inst 2007; 99:545–57.

90. Singh S, Singh AG, Singh PP, et al. Statins are associated with reduced risk of esophageal cancer, particularly in patients with Barrett's esophagus: a systematic review and meta-analysis. Clin Gastroenterol Hepatol 2013;11:620–9.

91. Nguyen T, Duan Z, Naik AD, et al. Statin use reduces risk of esophageal adenocarcinoma in US veterans with Barrett's esophagus: a nested case-control study. Gastroenterology 2015;149:1392–8.

92. Gaddam S, Singh M, Balasubramanian G, et al. Persistence of nondysplastic Barrett's esophagus identifies patients at lower risk for esophageal adenocarcinoma: results from a large multicenter cohort. Gastroenterology 2013; 145:548–53.e1.

93. Hur C, Choi SE, Rubenstein JH, et al. The cost effectiveness of radiofrequency ablation for Barrett's esophagus. Gastroenterology 2012;143:567–75.

94. Corley DA. Can you stop surveillance after radiofrequency ablation of Barrett's esophagus? A glass half full. Gastroenterology 2013;145:39–42.

95. Phoa KN, van Vilsteren FG, Weusten BL, et al. Radiofrequency ablation vs endoscopic surveillance for patients with Barrett esophagus and low-grade dysplasia: a randomized clinical trial. JAMA 2014;311:1209–17.

96. Sinh P, Anaparthy R, Young PE, et al. Clinical outcomes in patients with a diagnosis of "indefinite for dysplasia" in Barrett's esophagus: a multicenter cohort study. Endoscopy 2015;47:669–74.

97. Lim CH, Treanor D, Dixon MF, et al. Low-grade dysplasia in Barrett's esophagus has a high risk of progression. Endoscopy 2007;39:581–7.

98. Dulai GS, Shekelle PG, Jensen DM, et al. Dysplasia and risk of further neoplastic progression in a regional Veterans Administration Barrett's cohort. Am J Gastroenterol 2005;100:775–83.

99. Shaheen NJ, Crosby MA, Bozymski EM, et al. Is there publication bias in the reporting of cancer risk in Barrett's esophagus? Gastroenterology 2000;119: 333–8.

100. Dunbar KB, Spechler SJ. The risk of lymph-node metastases in patients with high-grade dysplasia or intramucosal carcinoma in Barrett's esophagus: a systematic review. Am J Gastroenterol 2012;107:850–62 [quiz: 863].

101. Shaheen NJ, Overholt BF, Sampliner RE, et al. Durability of radiofrequency ablation in Barrett's esophagus with dysplasia. Gastroenterology 2011;141:460–8.

102. Shaheen NJ, Sharma P, Overholt BF, et al. Radiofrequency ablation in Barrett's esophagus with dysplasia. N Engl J Med 2009;360:2277–88.

103. Gosain S, Mercer K, Twaddell WS, et al. Liquid nitrogen spray cryotherapy in Barrett's esophagus with high-grade dysplasia: long-term results. Gastrointest Endosc 2013;78:260–5.

104. Shaheen NJ, Greenwald BD, Peery AF, et al. Safety and efficacy of endoscopic spray cryotherapy for Barrett's esophagus with high-grade dysplasia. Gastrointest Endosc 2010;71:680–5.

105. Greenwald BD, Dumot JA. Cryotherapy for Barrett's esophagus and esophageal cancer. Curr Opin Gastroenterol 2011;27:363–7.

106. Leers JM, DeMeester SR, Oezcelik A, et al. The prevalence of lymph node metastases in patients with T1 esophageal adenocarcinoma a retrospective review of esophagectomy specimens. Ann Surg 2011;253:271–8.

107. Stein HJ, Feith M, Bruecher BL, et al. Early esophageal cancer: pattern of lymphatic spread and prognostic factors for long-term survival after surgical resection. Ann Surg 2005;242:566–73 [discussion: 573–5].

108. Buskens CJ, Westerterp M, Lagarde SM, et al. Prediction of appropriateness of local endoscopic treatment for high-grade dysplasia and early adenocarcinoma by EUS and histopathologic features. Gastrointest Endosc 2004;60:703–10.

109. Westerterp M, Koppert LB, Buskens CJ, et al. Outcome of surgical treatment for early adenocarcinoma of the esophagus or gastro-esophageal junction. Virchows Arch 2005;446:497–504.

110. Liu L, Hofstetter WL, Rashid A, et al. Significance of the depth of tumor invasion and lymph node metastasis in superficially invasive (T1) esophageal adenocarcinoma. Am J Surg Pathol 2005;29:1079–85.

111. Badreddine RJ, Prasad GA, Lewis JT, et al. Depth of submucosal invasion does not predict lymph node metastasis and survival of patients with esophageal carcinoma. Clin Gastroenterol Hepatol 2010;8:248–53.

112. Rice TW, Falk GW, Achkar E, et al. Surgical management of high-grade dysplasia in Barrett's esophagus. Am J Gastroenterol 1993;88:1832–6.
113. Heitmiller RF, Redmond M, Hamilton SR. Barrett's esophagus with high-grade dysplasia. An indication for prophylactic esophagectomy. Ann Surg 1996;224: 66–71.
114. Nigro JJ, Hagen JA, DeMeester TR, et al. Occult esophageal adenocarcinoma: extent of disease and implications for effective therapy. Ann Surg 1999;230: 433–8 [discussion: 438–40].
115. van Lanschot JJ, Hulscher JB, Buskens CJ, et al. Hospital volume and hospital mortality for esophagectomy. Cancer 2001;91:1574–8.

Management

Staging in Esophageal and Gastric Cancers

Thomas Hayes, MB ChB[a,b,c], Elizabeth Smyth, MB BCh, MSc[a,b,c,*],
Angela Riddell, MD[a,b,c], William Allum, MD[a,b,c]

KEYWORDS

• Gastric cancer • Esophageal cancer • Staging • PET • CT • MRI • Laparoscopy

KEY POINTS

• Accurately determining tumor stage before the commencement of treatment is vital for ensuring optimal outcomes for patients who will undergo surgical resection for gastro-esophageal cancer.
• All patients should undergo computerized tomography in the first instance to establish TNM stage, and PET should be used to detect occult metastases in patients with >T1/N1 or T2 tumors.
• For gastric cancers and distal esophageal cancers being considered for curative resection, laparoscopy ± peritoneal lavage should be performed.

INTRODUCTION

Gastric and esophageal cancers (OGCs) represent the fourth and seventh most common malignancies worldwide, with an estimated 631,300 and 323,000 new cases globally in 2012. The prognosis of patients diagnosed with esophagogastric cancer is notoriously poor, with modest outcomes seen from current treatments. Late presentation is a common feature of both diseases, with approximately half of esophageal tumors and up to 65% of patients with gastric cancer displaying locally advanced or metastatic disease at the time of diagnosis. Consequently, survival outcomes are disappointing, with less than 15% of patients alive 10 years postdiagnosis.[1–3]

The treatment options for esophagogastric cancers vary widely depending on both the site of the lesion and the stage of disease at presentation. Early tumors involving

Disclosure Statement: E. Smyth discloses honoraria for advisory board participation for Five Prime Therapeutics for an advisory role for Bristol-Myers Squibb. The other authors do not declare any disclosures.
[a] Department of Gastrointestinal Oncology, Royal Marsden Hospital, Fulham Road, London, SW3 6JJ, UK; [b] Department of Radiology, Royal Marsden Hospital, Fulham Road, London, SW3 6JJ, UK; [c] Department of Surgery, Royal Marsden Hospital, Fulham Road, London, SW3 6JJ, UK
* Corresponding author. Royal Marsden Hospital, Fulham Road, London, SW3 6JJ, UK.
E-mail address: Elizabeth.smyth@rmh.nhs.uk

Hematol Oncol Clin N Am 31 (2017) 427–440
http://dx.doi.org/10.1016/j.hoc.2017.02.002
0889-8588/17/© 2017 Elsevier Inc. All rights reserved.

hemonc.theclinics.com

only the superficial layers of the gastric or esophageal wall can be successfully cured by endoscopic mucosal resection (EMR) alone. More advanced disease may require aggressive preoperative and/or postoperative chemotherapy or chemoradiotherapy, in conjunction with radical surgery, which itself carries a significant risk of morbidity and mortality. Although some early squamous cell carcinoma may be cured using chemoradiotherapy, for adenocarcinoma patients, only surgery offers the prospect of cure, and even after adequate oncologic resection, recurrence is common. For patients with metastatic disease, such arduous treatment strategies confer no benefit, and extensive surgery with curative intent is inappropriate. In these cases, systemic chemotherapy alone represents best practice.

Consequently, it is self-evident that establishing an accurate tumor stage before the commencement of treatment is vital if potentially curable patients are to avoid being denied access to appropriate treatment. Similarly, inaccurate understaging may lead to inappropriate strategies being pursued with no realistic prospect of survival benefit to justify the associated morbidity and mortality. Precise local staging (T stage) identifies those patients suitable for endoscopic resection, whereas for more advanced tumors, this information, in conjunction with an assessment of nodal status and depth of local invasion, helps guide the appropriateness of adjuvant and neoadjuvant chemoradiotherapy. Such oncologic treatments have a role in gaining regional control over tumor spread and aid in securing adequate resection margins. The presence of distant metastases implies that such local control is impossible and usually renders surgical resection unjustified.

In this context, it is concerning that the modalities used to determine the cancer stage in such patients are regularly demonstrated to be inaccurate, and that much debate exists around the most appropriate strategies by which patients may be accurately staged. This review examines the investigations used in the staging of OGCs, including endoscopic ultrasound (EUS), computerized tomography (CT), MRI, and PET-CT. It summarizes their advantages and limitations, before progressing to consider appropriate strategies through which the pursuit of an accurate diagnosis may be achieved. It also considers the role of surgical diagnostic laparoscopy and its contribution to staging.

STAGING OF GASTRIC AND ESOPHAGEAL TUMORS

OGCs are staged by the TNM system, which defines their tumor stage from I to IV based on pathologic criteria.[4,5] Detailed descriptions of these staging criteria are listed in **Tables 1–3**, **Fig. 1**. The TNM classification ascribes a tumor stage based on the depth of invasion through the esophageal or gastric wall. The extent of lymph node metastases contributes the N stage, whereas more extensive lymphatic disease beyond the immediate nodal drainage basin in the context of esophageal cancer, or beyond regional lymph nodes in gastric cancer, is considered metastatic disease.

CANCER OF THE GASTROESOPHAGEAL JUNCTION

Gastroesophageal junction (GOJ) cancers behave differently than lower esophageal cancers and have been classified on clinical criteria into 3 types by Siewert and Stein.[6] Type I tumors arise from 1 to 5 cm proximal to the GOJ and may be considered tumors of the lower esophagus. Distal to this, type II tumors arise from 1 cm proximal to 2 cm distal to the GOJ and represent cardia carcinomas. Type III tumors arise from 2 to 5 cm distal to the GOJ and are also considered to be subcardial gastric carcinomas.

Table 1
Cancer staging categories for cancer of the esophagus and esophagogastric junction

Category	Criteria
T category	
TX	Tumor cannot be assessed
T0	No evidence of primary tumor
Tis	High-grade dysplasia, defined as malignant cells confined by the basement membrane
T1	Tumor invades the lamina propria, muscularis mucosae, or submucosa
T1a[a]	Tumor invades the lamina propria or muscularis mucosae
T1b[a]	Tumor invades the submucosa
T2	Tumor invades the muscularis propria
T3	Tumor invades the adventitia
T4	Tumor invades adjacent structures
T4a[a]	Tumor invades the pleura, pericardium, azygos vein, diaphragm, or peritoneum
T4b[a]	Tumor invades other adjacent structures, such as the aorta, vertebral body, or trachea
N category	
NX	Regional lymph nodes cannot be assessed
N0	No regional lymph node metastasis
N1	Metastasis in 1–2 regional lymph nodes
N2	Metastasis in 3–6 regional lymph nodes
N3	Metastasis in $\geq$7 regional lymph nodes
M category	
M0	No distant metastasis
M1	Distant metastasis
Adenocarcinoma G category	
GX	Differentiation cannot be assessed
G1	Well differentiated, with >95% of the tumor composed of well-formed glands
G2	Moderately differentiated, with 50%–95% of the tumor showing gland formation
G3[b]	Poorly differentiated, with tumors composed of nest and sheets of cells with <50% of the tumor demonstrating glandular formation
Squamous cell carcinoma G category	
GX	Differentiation cannot be assessed
G1	Well-differentiated, with prominent keratinization with pearl formation and a minor component of nonkeratinizing basal-like cells, tumor cells arranged in sheets, and mitotic counts low
G2	Moderately differentiated, with variable histologic features ranging from parakeratotic to poorly keratinizing lesions and pearl formation generally absent
G3[c]	Poorly differentiated, consisting predominantly of basal-like cells forming large and small nests with frequent central necrosis and with the nests consisting of sheets or pavement-like arrangements of tumor cells that are occasionally punctuated by small numbers of parakeratotic or keratinizing cells

(*continued on next page*)

Category	Criteria
Table 1 **(*continued*)**	
Category	**Criteria**
Squamous cell carcinoma L category[d]	
LX	Location unknown
Upper	Cervical esophagus to lower border of the azygos vein
Middle	Lower border of the azygos vein to lower border of the inferior pulmonary vein
Lower	Lower border of the inferior pulmonary vein to the stomach, including the esophagogastric junction

[a] Subcategories.
[b] If further testing of "undifferentiated" cancers reveals a glandular component, categorize as adenocarcinoma G3.
[c] If further testing of "undifferentiated" cancers reveals a squamous cell component or if after further testing they remain undifferentiated, categorize as squamous cell carcinoma G3.
[d] Location is defined by epicenter of esophageal tumor.
From Rice TW, Ishwaran H, Ferguson MK, et al. Cancer of the esophagus and esophagogastric junction: an eighth edition staging primer. J Thorac Oncol 2017;12(1):36–42.

Table 2 **TNM gastric cancer staging**	
Primary tumor (T)	
TX	Primary tumor cannot be assessed
T0	No evidence of primary tumor
Tis	Carcinoma in situ: intraepithelial tumor without invasion of the lamina propria
T1	Tumor invades lamina propria, muscularis mucosae, or submucosa
T1a	Tumor invades lamina propria or muscularis mucosae
T1b	Tumor invades submucosa
T2	Tumor invades muscularis propria
T3	Tumor penetrates subserosal connective tissue without invasion of visceral peritoneum or adjacent structures
T4	Tumor invades serosa (visceral peritoneum) or adjacent structures
T4a	Tumor invades serosa (visceral peritoneum)
T4b	Tumor invades adjacent structures
Regional lymph nodes (N)	
NX	Regional lymph node(s) cannot be assessed
N0	No regional lymph node metastasis
N1	Metastasis in 1–2 regional lymph nodes
N2	Metastasis in 3–6 regional lymph nodes
N3	Metastasis in 7 or more regional lymph nodes
N3a	Metastasis in 7–15 regional lymph nodes
N3b	Metastasis in 16 or more regional lymph nodes
Distant metastasis (M)	
M0	No distant metastasis
M1	Distant metastasis

Modified from Washington K. 7th edition of the AJCC cancer staging manual: stomach. Ann Surg Oncol 2010;17:3078; with permission.

Table 3			
Stage grouping of gastric cancer			
Stage	T	N	M
0	Tis	N0	M0
IA	T1	N0	M0
IB	T2	N0	M0
	T1	N1	M0
IIA	T3	N0	M0
	T2	N1	M0
	T1	N2	M0
IIB	T4a	N0	M0
	T3	N1	M0
	T2	N2	M0
	T1	N3	M0
IIIA	T4a	N1	M0
	T3	N2	M0
	T2	N3	M0
IIIB	T4b	N0	M0
	T4b	N1	M0
	T4a	N2	M0
	T3	N3	M0
IIIC	T4b	N2	M0
	T4b	N3	M0
	T4a	N3	M0
IV	Any T	Any N	M1

Modified from Washington K. 7th edition of the AJCC cancer staging manual: stomach. Ann Surg Oncol 2010;17:3078; with permission.

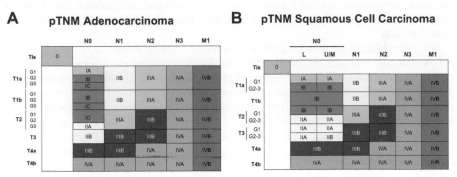

Fig. 1. (*A*) Pathologic stage groups (pTNM) of esophageal tumours: adenocarcinoma. (*B*) Pathologic stage groups (pTNM) of esophageal tumours: squamous cell carcinoma.

STAGING INVESTIGATIONS

The principal forms of staging investigations for OGCs are EUS, CT, MRI, and PET-CT. In addition, surgical diagnostic laparoscopy has a role to play in establishing the extent of disease and in contributing to treatment planning.

ENDOSCOPIC ULTRASOUND AND ENDOSCOPIC RESECTION

EUS assesses the depth of local tumor invasion as well as regional lymph node involvement. Although EUS can be extended to investigate the extent of metastatic disease within the abdomen, notably the presence of liver metastases and ascites, its primary role is as an indicator of the local-regional extent of disease and thus the feasibility of adequate surgical resection. One particular purported benefit of EUS is the ability to distinguish tumor invasion through the different layers of the esophageal or gastric wall and consequently to make an estimation of the tumor's T stage. In addition, EUS also offers the opportunity to interrogate suspicious lymph nodes through fine needle biopsy. Both these factors are important when considering whether EMR is feasible.[7]

EUS can take the form of an echoendoscope or used as a miniature ultrasound catheter deployed via a traditional esophagogastric endoscope. Echoendoscopes can be linear, offering a limited field of view in the same plane as the ultrasound transducer, or radial, affording 360° circumferential views of targets perpendicular to the scope. Both are considered to deliver similar performance; however, radial scopes may be preferred for tumor staging, and linear for fine needle aspiration (FNA) sampling.[8] The use of ultrasound catheters affords images with ultrahigh-frequency imaging, which gives better resolution of images at the expense of depth of penetration.[9] Deployment of miniature ultrasound catheters can also permit investigation of stricturing lesions without the need for dilatation and the attendant risk of perforation.

EMR can be considered for early tumors such as those staged as Tis (in situ) or T1N0. EMR is potentially curative while also contributing a method through which early neoplasia can be staged histologically. The depth of endoscopic resection is usually into the submucosa, and thus, submucosal invasion can be detected through histologic analysis. Therefore EMR represents the best method of assessment and proves superior to EUS, with a proven influence on subsequent management plans.[10–12] Submucosa is present in 88% of endoscopic resection samples compared with 1% of biopsy samples, with nearly all specimens containing lamina propria. Furthermore, EMR samples demonstrate greater interobserver agreement and assessment than FNA biopsy ones, making EMR preferable to EUS and FNA as a staging investigation for early malignancies.[13]

The widespread use of both EUS and EMR is however limited by many practical considerations. Perhaps more than any other staging modality, both are severely operator dependent. Significant technical skill is required to deploy probes appropriately and traverse stricturing lesions. Consequently, UK guidelines recommend EUS only be performed in centers with at least one trained endosonographer and a throughput of at least 100 patients annually.[14] Moreover, EUS and EMR are invasive procedures with significant scope for morbidity and even mortality. Perforation rates, particularly if dilation of a structuring lesion is undertaken, may approach 1%. Thus, it is recommended that the use of EUS is restricted to centers with the capability to manage such complications, and if needs be, perform emergency surgery.[8]

In addition, differences in technology between departments and the limitations imposed by a high degree of operator dependence have produced notable variation in the results reported from EUS. A recent meta-analysis of EUS performance in gastric cancer staging showed a pooled accuracy for T-stage diagnosis of 75%, with individual studies reporting rates from 56.9% to 87.7%.[15] A slight trend, although not statistically significant, was observed for better performance with increasing T stage. Although at its worst, one study reported that EUS only correctly identified T1 lesions 14% of the time, other studies reported up to 100% concordance between EUS findings and histology for all T stages. EUS has also been identified as struggling to distinguish T2 and T3 lesions where local inflammation can be mistaken for tumor invasion.

In relation to N staging, the same meta-analysis reported that EUS could under the best circumstances prove highly accurate with good sensitivity and specificity, although overall pooled results were less encouraging. EUS diagnostic accuracy for N staging ranged from 30% to 90%; sensitivity from 16.6% to 96.8%; and specificity from 57.1% to 100%. The pooled accuracy for N staging was 64% (95% confidence interval [CI]: 43%–84%); pooled sensitivity 74% (95% CI: 66%–81%); and pooled specificity 80% (95% CI: 74%–87%). No association was found between the performance of EUS as a staging modality and the technology used or case load of the department.

For tumors of the esophagus, Findlay and colleagues[16] report that 49 of 128 patients with T1 disease suggested on CT had the stage confirmed on EUS. However, of those staged as T2-T4a by CT, only 2 of 501 were found at EUS to have T1 disease. Consequently, although EUS may have a role in confirming a T1 diagnosis made provisionally on CT, it may contribute little to change management in patients whose CT suggested more advanced disease. For those identified on CT as T4b, 38% were confirmed on EUS and 45% refuted, potentially opening the prospect of surgical resection to those overstaged by CT. Given these findings though, EUS altered management in only 0.4% of patients staged as T2-T4a on CT. When the risk of perforation was considered, they recommended EUS be reserved for clarifying the true extent of disease in those thought to have T1 or T4b disease on CT. They did however identify a subgroup of patients with T2-T4a disease on CT who subsequently underwent PET and were found to have a maximum standardized uptake value (SUVmax) less than 6.38 and a fluoro-2-deoxy-D-glucose (FDG) avid length less than 3.4 cm. These patients had a 1 in 20 chance of demonstrating T1 disease on EUS. Given the significant prognostic and therapeutic implications of a T1 diagnosis, they recommended EUS for this specific subgroup to identify patients amenable to EMR (**Figs. 2** and **3**).

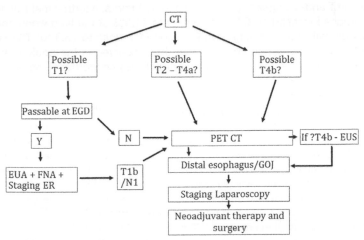

Fig. 2. Suggested algorithm for esophageal cancer. EGD, esophagogastroduodenoscopy; ER endoscopic resection; EUS, endoscopic ultrasound; N, no; Y, yes. (*Modified from* Findlay JM, Bradley KM, Maile EJ, et al. Pragmatic staging of oesophageal cancer using decision theory involving selective endoscopic ultrasonography, PET and laparoscopy. Br J Surg 2015;102(12):1496; with permission.)

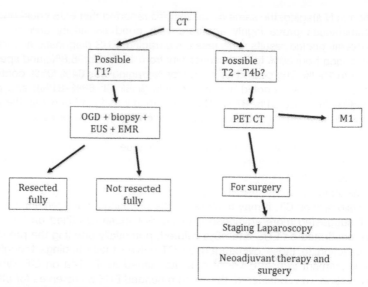

Fig. 3. Suggested algorithm for gastric cancer.

COMPUTERIZED TOMOGRAPHY

One principal aim of staging is the identification of distant metastatic disease. In the context of gastric or esophageal carcinoma, such patients are considered incurable by surgical resection and thus may embark on a separate treatment regimen with non-curative intent. Traditionally, establishing this "M stage" has used whole-body CT scanning to look for metastatic deposits in the chest, abdomen, or pelvis.

In addition to assessing the status of metastases, CT scanning also provides information on the T and N stages of gastroesophageal tumors. A further meta-analysis reported T stages identified on CT to be accurate 71.5% of the time when compared with histology, with rates varying from 63% for T1 lesions to 75.3 for T3 disease.[17] This represents a poorer performance than that observed in the pooled results for EUS. Furthermore, at its best no study reported 100% concordance between histology and CT, as was observed with EUS.

It is noteworthy that the use of multidetector CT enabling volumetric data acquisition has improved delineation of the primary tumor, with the ability to produce multiplanar reformat images. Upon further analysis, CT scanners with 4 or more detectors demonstrated an overall accuracy of 80%, with stage-specific accuracies of 75% to 84.5%.[17] The phenomenon by which T-staging accuracy is improved by the use of CT scanners with an increased number of detectors and through the use of multiplanar reformation of images is increasingly well documented. Consequently, recommendations have been made that they should be used in preference to single-detector scanners when assessing the T stage of gastric and esophageal tumors.[17–19]

In contrast to their findings regarding T-stage identification, Seevaratnam and colleagues[17] did not identify any improved performance from the use of increased detector numbers or multiplanar reconstruction images when assessing nodal or metastasis status by CT scanning. In particular, nodal assessment remains a diagnostic challenge, with their study suggesting that CT performed best when assessed by overall accuracy in comparison to findings at histology (66%), but enjoyed neither the sensitivity of MRI nor the specificity of PET scanning. Accuracy of nodal assessment particularly important because of the prognostic importance of nodal involvement and its influence on treatment. As neither CT nor MRI, by virtue of their noninvasive nature, permits histologic examination of lymph nodes, the determination of the significance of lymphadenopathy identified on radiological assessment relies on size criteria. Therefore CT and MRI assessment with it an inherent risk of understaging small metastatic deposits, while placing undue emphasis on reactive nodes. For M-stage analysis, CT scanning remains the mainstay of assessment and offers good accuracy, correctly identifying the M stage 82% of the time.

One point of controversy in the use of CT scanning relates to the reproducibility of CT protocols between departments. Again, this compromises any meta-analysis by introducing a substantial degree of heterogeneity across the studies involved. Seevaratnam and colleagues identified widespread variation in scanning technology, patient volumes, the subspecialty of radiologists, and scanning protocols, with oral and intravenous contrasts being used in different manners across the studies examined. Although no trends were observed in relation to the protocol used, it is clear that consensus is lacking over the best way in which CT scans should be executed.

MRI

MRI scans are increasingly used in the staging of gastrointestinal tumors because of their good soft tissue resolution. Although for cancers of the rectum, pelvic MRI assessment of tumor extent and local lymph node involvement represents the gold standard for regional staging, its use in upper gastrointestinal tract malignancies is a relatively new development with promising, albeit less developed evidence supporting its use. MRI has been shown in small single-center research studies to be of value in local staging of both esophageal and gastric cancers.[20,21] However, the main role in which MRI is currently used in the context of esophagogastric cancer is in the further characterization of focal liver lesions identified on other forms of cross-sectional imaging.

Although only 3 studies were identified pertaining to the use of MRI in gastric cancer staging, Seevaratnam and colleagues[17] report that MRI exceeds all other imaging modalities in demonstrating better agreement with histologic T staging. Overall, MRI was shown in the limited studies identified (involving only 109 patients) to enjoy an accuracy of 83%, with T stage–specific accuracies ranging from 77% to 87%. Although these results appear superficially encouraging, the small number and nature of the studies described open them to potential allegations of reporting bias. It is more than possible that as the use of MRI staging becomes more widespread, issues with the acceptability of MRI protocols to patients and the reproducibility of results across larger, non–study populations may become apparent. Although the large evidence basis underpinning the use of CT is likely demonstrative of its real world applicability, the small number of recruits to studies currently describing the use of MRI may disguise the influence of factors such as the need to use breath-holding protocols when scanning. As its use becomes more widespread, further studies will be needed to clarify its true efficiency in comparison to EUS and CT for the assessment of local T stage and nodal involvement.

PET-COMPUTERIZED TOMOGRAPHY

The use of 2-18F-FDG–labeled CT scans has increasingly become widespread in cancer staging. PET-CT works by combining the anatomic landmarks identified through traditional CT scanning with an assessment of the metabolic activity of various tissues made via their uptake of radiologically labeled glucose. Its usefulness however has been shown to vary by tumor site and type.

Generally, it can be considered that PET-CT offers low-resolution images, making it relatively unhelpful in the estimation of the degree of invasion by tumor of the gastric or esophageal wall or the presence of small volume lymphadenopathy, the latter of which can often be obscured by uptake from the adjacent primary. Its strength, however, is thought to lie in its detection of metastatic disease and as a guide to the response to neoadjuvant chemotherapy.

Specifically, in relation to gastric tumors, the reported pooled sensitivity for primary tumor detection afforded by PET-CT was estimated by Seevaratnan and colleagues[17] to be 80%, albeit from an evidence base limited to 3 studies. The reported sensitivity of PET scanning unsurprisingly increased with T stage, from 83% to 100% for T3/4 disease, versus 26% to 63% for T1 and T2 tumors.

PET-CT displays the lowest sensitivity for gastric cancer N stage (40%), although the highest specificity (98%). Consequently, PET-CT has a role in characterizing indeterminate lesions seen on CT, such as lung nodules. In addition, PET-CT demonstrated the highest accuracy when identifying distant metastases (88%), greater than higher-resolution CT scanning. PET-CT may also play an important role in detecting CT occult metastases in patients with operable gastric cancer; in one study of 113 patients with gastric cancer, 10% of patients were upstaged using PET-CT, whereas in a prospective Korean study, PET changed the management of 15% of patients with gastric cancer recruited.[22,23] However, it is noteworthy that the capacity of PET scanning to detect tumors varies by tumor type, with nonintestinal and signet ring carcinomas displaying a poor detectability by FDG-PET.[24]

Last, PET-CT in gastric cancer shows a good correlation between changes in the SUV after administration of neoadjuvant chemotherapy and the likelihood of tumor response. Therefore PET-CT allows the potential benefit of neoadjuvant therapy to be evaluated, with nonresponders identified early and treatment modified accordingly. Treatment success as measured by a decline in the SUV has also been shown to indicate long-term prognosis, making PET a useful adjunct in those undergoing neoadjuvant treatment.[25]

The role of PET-CT scanning in esophageal cancer varies somewhat from that in gastric cancer. Although it demonstrates the same limitations for T staging, it displays superior sensitivity and specificity than multidetector CT scanning for N stage. Furthermore, PET-CT scanning in esophageal cancer retains the strong ability to identify distant metastasis seen in gastric cancer. Consequently, Chowdhury and colleagues[26] report that PET-CT may influence management in as many as 40% of patients with esophageal cancer, principally in identifying those with metastatic disease unable to benefit from surgical resection. These findings mimic the important role observed by Findlay and colleagues,[16] who reported that PET-CT identified occult metastases in 14.9% of patients and changed management in 23%, although they noted that no patient with T1 disease on EUS was found to have metastases on the basis of PET-CT and thus questioned its use in this group. Such conclusions were echoed by another large series of PET-CT scans in patients with resectable esophageal cancer where PET-CT identified occult metastases in 13.6% of patients. In this series, when patients were blindly allocated into "high-risk" and "low-risk" groups, no patient in the low-risk group was upstaged using PET.[27]

In a similar manner to gastric cancer, changes in SUV levels associated with neoadjuvant therapy in esophageal cancer may indicate pathologic response. However, at present no consensus exists to the degree of SUV change required to identify nonresponders or when best to measure this, limiting its capacity to guide treatment strategies definitively.

STAGING LAPAROSCOPY

Diagnostic laparoscopy can be used in the staging of gastric cancers and distal esophageal cancers. Despite the best efforts of radiological staging, there remains considerable scope for inaccurate preoperative staging and a failure to detect the widespread disseminated peritoneal disease, which renders the patient incurable by surgical resection.[28] Such patients may then find themselves exposed to laparotomy with the intention of performing a curative surgical resection, which is immediately aborted upon initial inspection of the peritoneal cavity. This unnecessary surgical procedure carries with it significant morbidity and mortality.

In response to this, many promulgate the use of staging laparoscopy to ascertain the presence of disseminated peritoneal disease, which remains undetected by radiological methods. However, although the presumed stage of disease may be changed based on operative findings as frequently as 50% of the time, the use of surgical staging is by no means universal.[29,30]

Leake and colleagues[31] report that staging laparoscopy was moderately reliable in determining T or N stages compared with final histology. However, with regards to M staging, laparoscopy consistently demonstrated high levels of accuracy, sensitivity, and specificity, with respective reported values of 85% to 98.9%, 64.3% to 94%, and 80% to 100% in the studies included in their meta-analysis. Furthermore, they report that staging laparoscopy altered treatment in 8.5% to 59.6% of patients, with 8.5% to 43.8% of cases subsequently avoiding laparotomy. This finding would appear to support other studies such as Muntean and colleagues,[31,32] who assert that not only is diagnostic laparoscopy a beneficial tool for staging but also that by its influence, surgical treatment plans avoid unnecessary laparotomy. Perhaps unsurprisingly, cancers identified as early T-stage disease on radiological imaging enjoyed substantially less benefit from the procedure than those with locally advanced disease. In this regard, it may be that diagnostic laparoscopy is of greatest value in confirming or excluding the presence of incurable disease in those identified radiologically as being at the greatest risk.

In addition, staging laparoscopy affords the surgeon the opportunity to examine the peritoneal cavity for microscopic metastasis in the form of intraperitoneal free cancer cells (IFCC) through either the direct aspiration of ascitic fluid or the use of peritoneal lavage. Although the presence of such cells is widely accepted to be a poor prognostic indicator, it is unclear how the finding of free cells in the peritoneum should influence treatment, for instance, through the discontinuation of surgical resection or the use of intraperitoneal chemotherapy.[33] Nath and colleagues[34] report that the use of peritoneal lavage changed management in 7% of patients, namely, in the identification of those without overt peritoneal deposits or locally advanced tumors who already had microscopic peritoneal metastases. Consequently, they suggested that the presence of IFCCs guide the use of intraperitoneal chemotherapy at the time of laparoscopy, given a reported mean survival benefit of 15 months with its use compared with 9 months without.

SUMMARY
Esophageal Cancer

- CT should be used in the first instance to establish an approximate TNM stage.
- EUS in esophageal cancer should be reserved for patients with early disease and the potential for EMR or to distinguish T4a from T4b, where it influences management.
- PET should be used in esophageal cancer to identify occult metastasis in those patients with a local stage > T1/N1 or T2.

- Patients with esophageal or GOJ tumor being considered for curative resection should undergo laparoscopy ± peritoneal lavage.
- PET may have a helpful role in identifying responders and nonresponders to neoadjuvant therapy, although more evidence is required.
- MRI may be of benefit in determining local tumor stage, but evidence is so far confined to small numbers. Currently, its main use is in the characterization of indeterminate liver lesions seen on other staging investigations.

Gastric Cancer

- Again, CT represents the first staging investigation of choice.
- All patients should undergo an esophagogastroduodenoscopy, EUS, biopsy, and if appropriate, EMR.
- PET is likely superior to CT in identifying occult distal metastases and has a role in characterizing the response to neoadjuvant therapy.
- Staging laparoscopy should be undertaken for all patients undergoing curative resection for T3/T4 disease ± peritoneal lavage.
- MRI may be of benefit in determining local tumor stage, but evidence is so far confined to small numbers. Currently, its main use is in the characterization of indeterminate liver lesions seen on other staging investigations.

REFERENCES

1. Torre L, Bray F, Siegel R, et al. Global cancer statistics, 2012. CA Cancer J Clin 2015;65:87–108.
2. Casson AG, van Lanschot JJ. Recent advances in the management of esophageal adenocarcinoma. J Surg Oncol 2005;92:149–50.
3. Hundahl SA, Phillips JL, Menck HR. The national cancer data base report on poor survival of US gastric carcinoma patients treated with gastrectomy: fifth edition. American Joint committee on cancer staging, proximal disease, and the 'different disease' hypothesis. Cancer 2000;88:921–32.
4. Rice TW, Blackstone EH, Rusch V. 7th Edition of the AJCC; cancer staging manual; esophagus and esophagogastric junction. Ann Surg Oncol 2010;17: 1721–4.
5. Washington K. 7th edition of the AJCC cancer staging manual: stomach. Ann Surg Oncol 2010;17:3077–9.
6. Siewert JR, Stein HJ. Classification of adenocarcinoma of the esophagogastric junction. Br J Surg 1998;85:1457–9.
7. Bergman JJ, Fockens P. Endoscopic ultrasonography in patients with gastroesophageal cancer. Eur J Ultrasound 1999;10:127–38.
8. Penman I, NS, Harris K. Staging of oesophago-gastric carcinoma by endoscopic ultrasonography: guidance and minimum standards. UK EUS users group in association with the British society of Gastrienterology 2004.
9. Puli SR, Batapati Krishna Reddy J, Bechtold ML, et al. How good is endoscopic ultrasound for TNM staging of gastric cancer? A meta-analysis and systematic review. World J Gastroenterol 2008;14:4011–9.
10. Curver WL, Bansal A, Shrama P, et al. Endoscopic workup of early Barrett's neoplasia. Endoscopy 2008;40:1000–7.
11. Mino-Kenudson M, Hull MJ, Brown I, et al. EMR for Barrett's esophagus-related superficial neoplasms offers better diagnostic reproducibility than mucosal biopsy. Gastrointest Endosc 2007;66:660–6.

12. Peters FP, Brakehoff KP, Curvers WL, et al. Histologic evaluation of re-section specimens obtained at 293 endoscopic resections in Barrett'sesophagus. Gastrointest Endosc 2008;67:604–9.
13. Wani S, Mathur SC, Curvers WL, et al. Greater interobserver agreement by endoscopic mucosal resection than biopsy samples in Barrett's dysplasia. Clini Gastroenterol Hepatol 2010;8:783–8.
14. Allum WH, Blazeby JM, Griffin M, et al. Guidelines for the management of esophageal and gastric cancer. Gut 2011;60:1449–72.
15. Cardoso R, Coburn N, Seevaratnam R, et al. A systematic review and meta-analysis of the utility of EUS for preoperative staging for gastric cancer. Gastric Cancer 2012;15:19–26.
16. Findlay JM, Bradley KM, Maile EJ, et al. Pragmatic staging of oesophageal cancer using decision theory involving selective endoscopic ultrasonography, PET and laparoscopy. Br J Surg 2015;102:1488–99.
17. Seevaratnam R, Cardoso R, Mcgregor C, et al. How useful is preoperative imaging for tumor, node, metastasis (TNM) staging of gastric cancer? A meta-analysis. Gastric Cancer 2012;15:S3–18.
18. Chen CY, Wu DC, Kang WY, et al. Staging of gastric cancer with 16-channel MDCT. Abdom Imaging 2006;31:514–20.
19. Kim AY, Kim HJ, Ha HK. Gastric cancer by multidetector row CT: preoperative staging. Abdom Imaging 2005;30:465–72.
20. Albiin N. MRI of focal liver lesions. Curr Med Imaging Rev 2012;8:107–16.
21. Riddell AM, Allum WH, Thompson JN, et al. The appearances of esophageal carcinoma demonstrated on high-resolution, T2-weighted MRI, with histopathological correlation. Eur Radiol 2007;17:391–9.
22. Smyth E, Schöder H, Strong VE, et al. A prospective evaluation of the utility of 2-deoxy-2-[(18) F]fluoro-D-glucose positron emission tomography and computed tomography in staging locally advanced gastric cancer. Cancer 2012;15:5481–8.
23. Chen J, Cheong JH, Yun MJ, et al. Improvement in preoperative staging of gastric adenocarcinoma with positron emission tomography. Cancer 2005;103:2383–90.
24. Mukai K, Ishida Y, Okajima K, et al. Usefulness of preoperative FDG-PET for detection of gastric cancer. Gastric Cancer 2006;9:192–6.
25. Dassen AE, Lips DJ, Hoekstra CJ, et al. FDG-PET has no definite role in preoperative imaging in gastric cancer. Eur J Surg Oncol 2009;35:449–55.
26. Chowdhury FU, Bradley KM, Gleeson FV. The role of 18F-FDG PET/CT in the evaluation of oesophageal carcinoma. Clin Radiol 2008;63:1297–309.
27. Bunting DM, Lai WW, Berrisford RG, et al. Positron emission tomography-computed tomography in oesophageal cancer staging: a tailored approach. World J Surg 2015;39:1000–7.
28. Mahadevan D, Sudirman A, Kandasami P, et al. Laparoscopic staging in gastric cancer: an essential step in its management. J Minim Access Surg 2010;6:111–3.
29. Schwarz RE. Factors influencing change of preoperative treatment intent in a gastrointestinal cancer practice. World J Surg Oncol 2007;5:32.
30. Karanicolas P, Elkin EB, Jacks L, et al. Staging laparoscopy in the management of gastric cancer: a population-based analysis. J Am Coll Surg 2011;213:644–51.
31. Leake PA, Cardoso R, Seevaratnam R, et al. A systematic review of the accuracy and indications for diagnostic laparoscopy prior to curative-intent resection of gastric cancer. Gastric Cancer 2012;15:S38–47.
32. Muntean V, Mihailov A, Iancu C, et al. Staging laparoscopy in gastric cancer. Accuracy and impact on therapy. J Gastrointestin Liver Dis 2009;18:189–95.

33. Pecqueux M, Fritzmann J, Adamu M, et al. Free intraperitoneal tumor cells and outcome in gastric cancer patients: a systematic review and meta-analysis. Oncotarget 2015;3:35564–78.

34. Nath J, Moorthy K, Taniere P, et al. Peritoneal lavage cytology in patients with oesophagogastric adenocarcinoma. Br J Surg 2008;95:721–6.

Management of Locally Advanced Gastroesophageal Cancer
Still a Multidisciplinary Global Challenge?

Salah-Eddin Al-Batran, MD[a],*, Sylvie Lorenzen, MD[b]

KEYWORDS

- Gastroesophageal cancer • Perioperative • Locally advanced • Chemotherapy

KEY POINTS

- Available data indicate that patients with clinical stage II or III adenocarcinoma of stomach, gastroesophageal junction (GEJ), and esophagus benefit from multimodality treatment approaches.
- Therapy options for western patients include perioperative chemotherapy for both gastric and GEJ cancer, postoperative chemoradiation for gastric cancer, and preoperative chemoradiation for esophageal adenocarcinoma.
- In terms of perioperative chemotherapy protocols, platinum-fluoropyrimidine doublets, such as cisplatin and 5-fluorouracil (5-FU) (CF); triplets, such as epirubicin, cisplatin, and capecitabine (ECX); or docetaxel, 5-FU, leucovorin, oxaliplatin, and docetaxel (FLOT) are appropriate regimens.
- Current studies still do not recommend a preferred chemotherapy regimen but rates of complete pathologic remission differ among the regimens and are approximately at 2% with CF, 7% with ECX, and 16% with FLOT.
- Adding postoperative radiotherapy to established perioperative or adjuvant protocols did not improve survival.
- Future studies will focus on evaluating the role of biologic agents such as trastuzumab and pertuzumab (for HER2-positive disease), or ramucirumab, as well as immunomodulatory antibodies, such as programmed death (PD)-1 or programmed death-ligand (PD-L1) antibodies.

Disclosure Statement: Advisory role - Merck, Roche, Celgene, Lilly, Nordic Pharma; Speaker - Roche, Celgene, Lilly, Nordic Pharma; Research grants - Sanofi, Roche, Celgene, Vifor, Medac, Hospira, Lilly (S.-E. Al-Batran). Advisory role - Eli-Lilly, Roche, Sanofi-Aventis; Speaker - Eli-Lilly, Merck, MSD; Research grants - Eli Lilly (S. Lorenzen).

[a] Institute of Clinical Cancer Research, Krankenhaus Nordwest, UCT-University Cancer Center, Steinbacher Hohl 2-26, Frankfurt am Main 60488, Germany; [b] Department of Hematology and Oncology, Klinikum rechts der Isar der TU München, Ismaninger Straße 22, München 81675, Germany
* Corresponding author.
E-mail address: albatran@aol.com

Hematol Oncol Clin N Am 31 (2017) 441–452
http://dx.doi.org/10.1016/j.hoc.2017.01.004
0889-8588/17/© 2017 Elsevier Inc. All rights reserved.

hemonc.theclinics.com

OVERVIEW AND INTRODUCTION

Although the overall gastric cancer incidence is decreasing, the incidence of adeno-carcinoma of the gastroesophageal junction (GEJ) has increased.[1] The global shift of gastric cancer (and esophageal cancer) location toward the GEJ[2,3] led the International Union Against Cancer (UICC) to adopt the GEJ cancers into its seventh edition of the tumor-node-metastasis (TNM) classification as a new entity.[4] These tumors were staged as esophageal tumors, triggering a new controversy, because cardia cancer and distal esophageal tumors are treated in a different way in many regions, particularly with regard to the surgical therapy.

The symptoms of gastroesophageal cancer appear relatively late. Therefore, most of affected individuals present with locally advanced disease; that is, with clinical stage of T3 or T4 and/or regional lymph nodes that are affected by disease, or even with distant metastases. As a result, gastric and GEJ carcinomas are commonly fatal diseases with 5-year survival rates of approximately 20% to 30%.[5,6] Surgery remains the only form of curative treatment but is associated with relatively high rates of regional and distant recurrence. Therefore, it has become a worldwide consensus that surgery alone is no longer the standard of care in the management of these tumors. Numerous multidisciplinary strategies have been evaluated during the last decades to improve the treatment results by adding adjuvant or neoadjuvant systemic therapy, sometimes combined with radiotherapy. These approaches resulted in an absolute improvement in survival of around 10% to 15% over surgery alone but have not been compared head-to-head in appropriately powered clinical trials. Therefore, the optimal therapeutic approach remains controversial and practices vary around the globe. This article summarizes the current evidence of various approaches, highlights some ongoing and planned clinical trials, and suggests options to further improve current treatment strategies and, thereby, prognosis of gastric and GEJ tumors.

DIFFERENCES WITHIN THE CATEGORIES GASTRIC, GASTRIC CARDIA, AND LOWER ESOPHAGEAL ADENOCARCINOMA: DOES LOCATION AND HISTOLOGY MATTER?

Besides the different anatomic regions and lymph node compartments affected by the tumor, substantial differences between gastric noncardia, gastric cardia, and lower esophageal adenocarcinomas exist. Tumors located in the cardia and distal esophagus are predominately intestinally differentiated, compared with the stomach cancers, where diffuse tumors are more commonly located. In terms of epidemiology, stomach cancers are more prevalent in Asian countries, whereas cardia cancer and distal esophageal adenocarcinomas are typically seen in the West (eg, Europe, North America, and South America). The groups are also distinct in terms of the underlying risk factors. Gastroesophageal reflux and consecutive Barrett metaplasia are the major risk factor associated with esophageal adenocarcinoma. This association could not be clearly established for gastric cardia cancer. For more distal stomach cancers, *Helicobacter pylori* infection and nutritional habits are well-recognized risk factors. In the metastatic setting, there is a general consensus that response and survival following chemotherapy is similar among the groups.[7] However, in curable patients, outcomes after surgical resection and response to perioperative chemotherapy are different.[8–12]

The Medical Research Council Adjuvant Gastric Infusional Chemotherapy (MAGIC)[13] and Fédération Nationale des Centres de Lutte contre le Cancer (FNCLCC)/Fédération Francophone de Cancérologie Digestive (FFCD)[14] studies were the first to show that the benefit from neoadjuvant chemotherapy seemed to be greater in GEJ tumors compared with gastric noncardia or true esophageal cancers. The hazard ratios (HRs) for death were particularly favorable in the GEJ subgroups in both studies and were at 0.57 (95% CI 0.39–0.83) and 0.49 (95% CI 0.28–0.88) in the MAGIC and FNCLCC/FFCD trials, respectively. This observation has been confirmed by a recent meta-analysis[12] and by recent studies demonstrating unexpectedly high rates of complete pathologic response (pathologic complete regression [pCR]) with neoadjuvant docetaxel-based triplet chemotherapy combinations.[10,11,15] In a pooled analysis of 3 German phase II studies of neoadjuvant or perioperative docetaxel-platinum-fluoropyrimidine triplets,[10] 18 of 120 (15%) subjects achieved a pCR. The pCR rate in subjects with junctional tumors compared with stomach cancer was 22% versus 6%, respectively (P = .019). These data support the concept that GEJ tumors may be preferentially treated with chemotherapy, given the higher rate of response to combination therapy regimens than that observed with tumors in distal esophagus or noncardia stomach.

Another consistent finding is that intestinal type tumors (according to Lauren classification) are more likely to achieve a pCR following preoperative chemotherapy compared with diffuse type tumors.[10,11,15] In the 5-FU, Leucovorin, Oxaliplatin, and Docetaxel (FLOT)-4 trial, the centrally assessed rate of pCR in subjects with gastric and GEJ cancers receiving perioperative 5-fluorouracil (5-FU), leucovorin, oxaliplatin, and docetaxel (FLOT) was 23% in the intestinal type subgroup and 3% in the diffuse type subgroup. Furthermore, a retrospective analysis has suggested that certain tumor histologies, specifically signet-ring cell or diffuse tumors, maybe be inherently resistant to standard chemotherapy regimens and, therefore, may not benefit from preoperative therapy,[16] although the analysis has to be interpreted with caution due to its retrospective nature.

Despite these substantial differences, all of the groups have been variably included in either esophageal or gastric cancer studies. Esophageal cancer studies have typically enrolled both squamous cell and adenocarcinoma histologies, 2 different diseases with dissimilar risk factors, prognosis, and even different staging according to American Joint Committee on Cancer (AJCC)/UICC classification.[4] Due to this heterogeneity, results of clinical trials are sometimes difficult to interpret. Researchers should, therefore, consider tumor histology and anatomic location when designing perioperative clinical trials in the future.

MULTIMODAL TREATMENT OPTIONS: IMPORTANCE OF CHEMOTHERAPY, RADIOTHERAPY, AND SURGERY
Perioperative Chemotherapy

In Europe and the United States, a predominant approach is to administer perioperative chemotherapy for resectable gastroesophageal cancer, based on the MAGIC trial. The MAGIC study[13] was the first trial to show an improvement of survival by perioperative chemotherapy in subjects with gastric, GEJ, and lower esophageal cancers. In this trial, conducted in the United Kingdom, 503 subjects with clinical stage II or III adenocarcinoma of the stomach (75%), GEJ (11.5%), and lower esophagus (14.5%) were either treated with 3 cycles of epirubicin, cisplatin, and 5-FU (ECF) presurgery and postsurgery, or surgery alone. The chemotherapy arm showed a statistically significant improvement in overall survival (OS) (5-year rates 36% vs 23%; HR 0.75, 95% CI 0.60–0.93, P = .009) compared with surgery alone. Few subjects (11%) in the MAGIC trial had GEJ cancers; however, this subgroup seemed to derive the highest benefit from chemotherapy (HR for death 0.49, 95% CI 0.28–0.88).

A similar degree of benefit was noted in the second landmark trial of perioperative chemotherapy, the French FNCLCC/FFCD 9703 study.[14] In contrast to all other adjuvant and perioperative trials, the FNCLCC/FFCD 9703 study trial was dominated by GEJ. Sixty-four percent of all 224 subjects enrolled had GEJ, 11% had lower esophageal tumors, and 24% had gastric adenocarcinoma. Subjects received 2 to 3 cycles of cisplatin–5-FU (CF) followed by surgery or surgery alone. After surgery, subjects in the chemotherapy arm who responded to the preoperative therapy received additional cycles of chemotherapy. Treatment with neoadjuvant or perioperative chemotherapy resulted in significantly improved OS (5-year OS rate 38% vs 24%; HR 0.69, 95% CI 0.50–0.95, P = .02). Similar to the MAGIC trial, the subgroup of GEJ tumors derived the highest benefit from perioperative chemotherapy (HR 0.57, 95% CI 0.39–0.83).

Since then, there have been intensive clinical research activities to further improve perioperative protocols. Most recently, results of the phase II part of the German FLOT4 phase III trial,[15] comparing the anthracycline-based triplet ECF with the docetaxel-based triplet FLOT in the perioperative setting, were presented (phase II, n = 300; phase III, n = 716).[15] In the study, resectable subjects with gastric (48%) or GEJ adenocarcinoma (52%) were randomly assigned to either 3 plus 3 cycles of perioperative ECF or epirubicin, cisplatin, and capecitabine (ECX) every 3 weeks or 4 plus 4 cycles of perioperative FLOT every 2 weeks. Primary endpoint of the phase II part was pCR (tumor regression grade [TRG]1a) assessed centrally according to Becker criteria.[17] FLOT was associated with significantly higher rates of pCR compared with ECF-ECX (16% vs 6%; P = .015). Also, the rate of complete or subtotal regression (TRG1a/b) was significantly higher with FLOT (37% vs 23%, P = .015). The differences were more pronounced in intestinal type tumors. Thirty-day mortality was 4% with ECF-ECX and 2% with FLOT (P = not significant [NS]). Postsurgical morbidity was 40% with ECF-ECX and 25% with FLOT (P = .02). Survival results of the Phase III FLOT4 trial will be presented at ASCO 2017.[15]

Another recent phase III trial (STO03) compared 3 plus 3 cycles of perioperative ECX with the same therapy plus bevacizumab followed by bevacizumab maintenance for subjects with potentially resectable gastric and GEJ adenocarcinoma. Progression-free survival and OS were similar between the study arms, as were the rates of pathologic remission, with a pCR rate of 5% and 7% for ECX and ECX plus bevacizumab, respectively, when the intention-to-treat population was used as the denominator.[8]

The randomized phase III OE05 trial compared 2 cycles of neoadjuvant CF with 4 cycles of neoadjuvant ECX followed by resection for lower esophageal and GEJ (types I and II) adenocarcinoma (n = 897). This study did not show a statistically significant improvement of OS (primary endpoint; HR 0.92, P = .302), although a trend for progression-free survival (P = .06), favoring 4 cycles of ECX, was seen.[18] Chemotherapy-related toxicity was higher with 4 cycles of ECX compared with 2 cycles of CF; however, surgical morbidity and mortality were similar.

Preoperative Chemoradiation

For esophageal cancer, neoadjuvant chemoradiation has become the standard of care in many countries based on several prospective trials and corresponding meta-analyses. Whether the data obtained in esophageal cancer can be extended to GEJ adenocarcinoma remains a controversial topic. The CROSS study was the most recent and largest trial to show a survival benefit from chemoradiation in esophageal cancer.[19] In this study, 366 subjects with squamous-cell carcinoma (23%) or adenocarcinoma of the esophagus (75%) were randomly assigned to chemotherapy with weekly paclitaxel and carboplatin combined with radiation therapy followed by surgery or to surgery alone. Only 24% percent of the total population had GEJ cancer. The median survival clearly favored neoadjuvant chemoradiation over surgery alone (HR 0.66, 95% CI 0.495–0.871, $P = .003$). The specific results for the GEJ subgroup were not presented; however, the adenocarcinoma group benefited less (HR 0.74, 95% CI 0.536–1.024, $P = .07$) than the squamous cell carcinoma group (HR 0.42, 95% CI 0.226–0.788, $P = .007$). With respect to early-stage esophageal cancer, it seems that there is no additional benefit of neoadjuvant chemoradiation over surgery alone. The French FFCD 9901 study[20] randomized predominantly stage I or II squamous-cell carcinoma subjects to surgery with or without preoperative chemoradiation. Three-year OS was similar in both study groups (chemoradiation, 47.5%; surgery alone, 53.0%; $P = .94$), whereas postoperative mortality rate increased (11.1% vs 3.4%; $P = .049$). The trial was stopped early for futility. Therefore, a neoadjuvant chemoradiation is not recommended for stage I esophageal cancer.

A smaller study that compared neoadjuvant induction chemotherapy followed by chemoradiation with chemotherapy alone in GEJ cancer was the German POET trial.[21] In this study, 126 subjects with adenocarcinoma of the lower esophagus or gastric cardia were randomly assigned to chemotherapy followed by surgery or chemotherapy followed by chemoradiation followed by surgery. The trimodality treatment improved pCR rates (15.6% vs 2%) and there was a statistical trend toward improved 3-year survival rates ($P = .07$).

Adjuvant Chemotherapy

Japanese and Korean adjuvant chemotherapy trials showed a clear benefit of adjuvant therapy for stage II or III gastric cancer using S1 administered orally for 1 year after surgery or intravenous capecitabine and oxaliplatin (XELOX).[22] However, European trials of adjuvant chemotherapy for gastric cancer have been disappointing so far. Three prospective trials evaluating postoperative chemotherapy compared with surgery alone showed 5-year survival rates ranging between 40% and 50%, with no significant differences between the arms.[23–25] A meta-analysis suggested a small survival benefit with adjuvant chemotherapy[26] that remained constant after testing for heterogeneity according to the geographic region where the study has been conducted (Europe, Asia, North America) and the regimen (monotherapy or combination chemotherapy) that has been given.

Adjuvant Chemoradiation

The only randomized prospective trial to support adjuvant (postoperative) chemoradiation for gastric and GEJ cancer is the Intergroup 116 trial.[27] In this trial, 556 subjects were randomly assigned to postoperative radiochemotherapy with bolus 5-FU and leucovorin and 45 Gy of radiation or surgery alone. Of note, only 20% of the subjects had GEJ tumors. Median survival for the entire population was improved from 27 to 36 months ($P = .005$) with chemoradiation, translating into a 3-year survival rate of 50% compared with 41% with surgery alone ($P = .005$), and an improved 3-year relapse-free survival rate of 48% versus 31% ($P = .001$) in favor for chemoradiation. After a median follow-up of 10.3 years, an OS benefit was maintained ($P = .005$).[28] Despite these positive results, the study was criticized for the low rate of D2 lymph node dissection, with 54% of subjects having less than a D1 or D2 resection, and because the survival rates in the Intergroup trial were not better than those observed in the negative European adjuvant trials.

A first attempt to answer the question of whether postoperative radiation is beneficial after D2 lymphadenectomy was made by the Korean Adjuvant Chemoradiation Therapy in Stomach Cancer (ARTIST) trial. In this trial, 458 subjects with stage Ib-IV

(M0) gastric cancer were randomized to either 6 cycles of adjuvant capecitabine-cisplatin or to 2 cycles of capecitabine-cisplatin before and after capecitabine-based chemoradiation.[29] The study was negative; however, a statically nonsignificant trend toward an improved 3-year disease-free survival (DFS) (78.2% vs 74.2%, $P = .09$) was noted with chemoradiation. In an unplanned subgroup analysis of 396 subjects with lymph-node positive disease, 3-year DFS was significantly improved with chemoradiation (77.5% vs 72.3%; $P = .04$). With a median follow-up of 7 years, the final report of the ARTIST trial still shows no significant difference in DFS and no difference in OS for the entire study population; however, the node-positive subjects treated on the chemoradiation arm still retain a DFS advantage.[30] As a consequence, a subsequent trial (ARTIST II) (ClinicalTrials.gov, NCT0176146) has been initiated to examine postoperative chemoradiation for subjects with lymph node–positive gastric cancer receiving D2 lymph node dissection.

Recently, the results from the Dutch multicenter, randomized, phase III CRITICS study (NCT00407186), which evaluated 3 cycles of preoperative ECX followed by gastrectomy and either 3 more cycles of postoperative ECX or chemoradiation with capecitabine-cisplatin, were presented. Subjects undergoing neoadjuvant chemotherapy followed by surgery with curative intent had similar progression-free and OS regardless of whether they received chemotherapy or chemoradiotherapy after surgery.[31]

OPTIONS TO IMPROVE CURRENT MULTIMODAL APPROACHES
Adaptive Therapy Based on Early Response Prediction

Since perioperative chemotherapy became standard in Europe for resectable gastro-esophageal cancer, both the accuracy of the pretherapeutic staging and the evaluation of response gained particular importance.[13,32] It is generally accepted that responders to chemotherapy have a significant improved survival compared with non-responders.[33] However, despite the proven benefit of neoadjuvant chemotherapy, less than half of the treated subjects respond to treatment. Currently, there are no established markers that can help to identify potential nonresponders at baseline or during the early phase of treatment.[34]

One option to early modify treatment according to response is the use of pretreatment and post-treatment 18-fluorodeoxyglucose (FDG) PET scans for early response assessment.

Previous results from the Metabolic response evaluatioN for Individualisation of neo-adjuvant Chemotherapy in Esophageal and esophagogastric adeNocarcinoma (MUNI-CON)-1[34] and MUNICON-2[35] trials have shown that PET-based therapy individualization is a feasible approach. The MUNICON-1 showed that subjects with a PET response, defined as a standardized uptake value decrease of 35% or more 2 weeks after induction therapy with CF, who continued chemotherapy for an additional 12 weeks had a significantly improved OS compared with PET-nonresponders who immediately proceeded to surgery.[34] This PET-guided treatment algorithm was evaluated in another trial, in which PET responders continued preoperative chemotherapy and nonresponders underwent salvage chemoradiation. Despite the addition of radiation therapy, margin-free resection (R0) rate and survival remained poor, which indicates a generally aggressive disease biology in primarily nonresponding subjects.[35] Shortcomings of PET-guided strategies include that the information gained by PET evaluation is prognostic rather than predictive. It is still hard to use the results to rationally modify the direction of therapeutic strategy. Moreover, response assessment with FDG-PET is limited to tumors located in the esophagus or GEJ and the intestinal type tumors, such as gastric cancers, and those of diffuse histology have limited FDG avidity.

Optimization by Targeted Therapy

HER-2–directed therapy improved survival in subjects with metastatic HER-2 positive gastric and GEJ adnocarcinoma,[36] and represents a promising predictive marker for HER-2–positive, early-stage disease. Based on the promising results of 2 perioperative, single-arm phase II studies with trastuzumab,[37,38] 2 randomized studies were initiated to assess the potential benefit of adding the HER-2 antibodies trastuzumab and pertuzumab to established perioperative therapy. The Arbeitsgemeinschaft Internistische Onkologie (AIO) (PETRARCA phase II/III study; NCT02581462) assigns subjects to perioperative FLOT with or without trastuzumab and pertuzumab. The 3-arm study by the European Organization for Research and Treatment of Cancer (EORTC) assigns subjects to perioperative cisplatin-capecitabine alone, or the same therapy with trastuzumab or trastuzumab and pertuzumab (INNOVATON phase II study; NCT02205047). Another key pathway involved in tumorigenesis is the angiogenic pathway. The use of the vascular endothelial growth factor receptor (VEGFR)- 2 antibody ramucirumab has added benefit in the second-line setting.[39,40] The phase II/III AIO RAMSES trial (NCT02661971) is addressing the value of ramucirumab in addition to FLOT chemotherapy in HER-2–negative gastric and GEJ adenocarcinoma. Furthermore, the RTOG 1010 trial is evaluating the additional benefit of trastuzumab to neoadjuvant chemoradiation with carboplatin-paclitaxel (NCT01196390).

In addition, immunotherapeutic strategies have shown early signs of efficacy in advanced chemorefractory disease.[8,41] Therefore, assessment of PD-1/PD-L1 inhibitors within the frame of multidisciplinary treatment may provide new opportunities for patients who have locally advanced gastroesophageal cancer.

SUMMARY

Treatment of locally advanced, resectable gastric, and GEJ cancer remains a challenge. Although several strategies improve prognosis, survival rates remain far from satisfactory. Optimized therapeutic strategies are needed, including the evaluation of targeted agents, novel regimens, and better chemotherapy or chemoradiation protocols and technics. The controversy regarding the role of radiation therapy can only be resolved in a well-powered phase III trial conducted with subjects with GEJ adenocarcinoma. Moreover, reliable methods for the prediction of response to neoadjuvant chemotherapy are needed. Imaging or other novel biomarkers could help to use response-directed treatment strategies to alter treatment of nonresponding patients to more effective therapies early in the course of treatment. Patients with poor response criteria may be candidates for a primary operation or may be treated with new drugs or intensified chemotherapy or chemoradiation schedules within clinical trials.

There are still open questions regarding the duration of preoperative chemotherapy and whether the postoperative component is necessary. Future studies should focus on the optimizing the postoperative therapy part. So far, the value of postoperative therapy guided by pathologic findings has not been assessed in randomized trials. Future studies also need to focus on GEJ and gastric cancer subjects as separate entities, to provide more robust data on both tumors. Future studies also need to pay more attention to the Lauren type of histology. Molecular markers for gastric cancer, such as HER2 or VEGFR could provide a basis to develop new treatment strategies. Because the PD-1 inhibitors, pembrolizumab (KEYNOTE 012) and nivolumab (CheckMate 032), have both shown activity in advanced gastric cancers, evaluating immunotherapies in the setting of early stage is of particular interest (**Table 1**).

Table 1
Selected perioperative phase III studies in localized esophagogastric cancer

Trial Acronym or Location of the Primary Cancer	Number in Subsample (n) for Histology	Design	R0 ITT[a]	pCR ITT[a]	5- or 3-y OS	OS Significantly Improved?
MAGIC[13] Stomach, 74% GEJ, 11% ES, 15%	n = 503 ADC	Perioperative 3 + 3 cycles ECF vs surgery alone	68% vs 66%	Not reported	5-y OS: 36% vs 23%	Yes
FFCD/ACCO[14] Stomach, 25% GEJ, 64% ES, 11%	n = 224 ADC	Perioperative 3 + 3 cycles CF vs surgery alone	84% vs 74%	Not reported	5-y OS: 38% vs 24%	Yes
EORTC 40954[32] Stomach, 49% GEJ, 51%	n = 144 ADC	Neoadjuvant CLF (2 cycles) vs surgery alone	82% vs 67%	7% vs NA	Not reported	No
AIO FLOT4[15] Stomach, 47% GEJ, 53%	n = 265 ADC	Perioperative 4 + 4 cycles FLOT vs perioperative 3 + 3 cycles ECF or ECX	85% vs 74%	16% vs 6%	—	NK yet
OE05[18] GEJ, nk ES, nk	n = 897 ADC	Neoadjuvant 4 cycles ECX vs neoadjuvant 2 cycles CF	50% vs 47%	7% vs 2%	3-y OS: 42% vs 39%	No

STO03[8] Stomach, 36% GEJ, 51% ES, 14%	n = 1063 ADC	Perioperative 3 + 3 cycles ECX + bevacizumab vs perioperative 3 + 3 cycles ECX	57% vs 59%	7% vs 5%	3-y OS: 48% vs 49%	No
POET[21] GEJ, 119	n = 119 ADC	Induction CT (15 wk) + surgery vs induction CT (12 wk) followed by CRT (3 wk) + surgery	72% vs 70%	16% vs 2%	3-y OS: 47% vs 28%	No (trend)
CROSS[19] GEJ, 24% ES, 76%	n = 366 ADC/SCC	Neoadjuvant CRT vs surgery alone	82% vs 59%	23% (ADC group) vs NA	5-y OS: 47% vs 34%	Yes

Abbreviations: ADC, adenocarcinoma; CLF, cisplatin, leucovorin, fu; CRT, chemoradiotherapy; CT, chemotherapy; GEJ, gastroesophageal junction; ITT, Intention-to-treat; NA, not applicable; NK, not known; ES, esophagus; SCC, squamous cell carcinoma.
[a] Percentages were recalculated using all randomized subjects as denominator.

REFERENCES

1. Botterweck AA, Schouten LJ, Volovics A, et al. Trends in incidence of adenocarcinoma of the oesophagus and gastric cardia in ten European countries. Int J Epidemiol 2000;29(4):645–54.
2. Simard EP, Ward EM, Siegel R, et al. Cancers with increasing incidence trends in the United States: 1999 through 2008. CA Cancer J Clin 2012;62(2):118–28.
3. Pohl H, Welch HG. The role of overdiagnosis and reclassification in the marked increase of esophageal adenocarcinoma incidence. J Natl Cancer Inst 2005; 97(2):142–6.
4. Rice TW, Blackstone EH, Rusch VW. 7th edition of the AJCC Cancer Staging Manual: esophagus and esophagogastric junction. Ann Surg Oncol 2010;17(7): 1721–4.
5. Devesa SS, Blot WJ, Fraumeni JF Jr. Changing patterns in the incidence of esophageal and gastric carcinoma in the United States. Cancer 1998;83(10): 2049–53.
6. Reim D, Loos M, Vogl F, et al. Prognostic implications of the seventh edition of the International Union Against Cancer classification for patients with gastric cancer: the Western experience of patients treated in a single-center European institution. J Clin Oncol 2013;31(2):263–71.
7. Chau I, Norman AR, Cunningham D, et al. Multivariate prognostic factor analysis in locally advanced and metastatic esophago-gastric cancer–pooled analysis from three multicenter, randomized, controlled trials using individual patient data. J Clin Oncol 2004;22(12):2395–403.
8. Cunningham D, Stenning SP, Smyth EC, et al. Peri-operative chemotherapy with or without bevacizumab in operable oesophagogastric adenocarcinoma (UK Medical Research Council ST03): primary analysis results of a multicentre, open-label, randomised phase 2-3 trial. Lancet Oncol 2017. http://dx.doi.org/ 10.1016/S1470-2045(17)30043-8.
9. Piso P, Werner U, Lang H, et al. Proximal versus distal gastric carcinoma–what are the differences? Ann Surg Oncol 2000;7(7):520–5.
10. Lorenzen S, Thuss-Patience P, Al-Batran SE, et al. Impact of pathologic complete response on disease-free survival in patients with esophagogastric adenocarcinoma receiving preoperative docetaxel-based chemotherapy. Ann Oncol 2013; 24(8):2068–73.
11. Homann N, Pauligk C, Luley K, et al. Pathological complete remission in patients with oesophagogastric cancer receiving preoperative 5-fluorouracil, oxaliplatin and docetaxel. Int J Cancer 2012;130(7):1706–13.
12. Ronellenfitsch U, Schwarzbach M, Hofheinz R, et al. Preoperative chemo(radio) therapy versus primary surgery for gastroesophageal adenocarcinoma: systematic review with meta-analysis combining individual patient and aggregate data. Eur J Cancer 2013;49(15):3149–58.
13. Cunningham D, Allum WH, Stenning SP, et al. Perioperative chemotherapy versus surgery alone for resectable gastroesophageal cancer. N Engl J Med 2006; 355(1):11–20.
14. Ychou M, Boige V, Pignon JP, et al. Perioperative chemotherapy compared with surgery alone for resectable gastroesophageal adenocarcinoma: an FNCLCC and FFCD multicenter phase III trial. J Clin Oncol 2011;29(13):1715–21.
15. Al-Batran SE, Hofheinz RD, Pauligk C, et al. Histopathological regression after neoadjuvant docetaxel, oxaliplatin, fluorouracil, and leucovorin versus epirubicin, cisplatin, and fluorouracil or capecitabine in patients with resectable gastric or

gastro-oesophageal junction adenocarcinoma (FLOT4-AIO): results from the phase 2 part of a multicentre, open-label, randomised phase 2/3 trial. Lancet Oncol 2016;17(12):1697–708.

16. Messager M, Lefevre JH, Pichot-Delahaye V, et al. The impact of perioperative chemotherapy on survival in patients with gastric signet ring cell adenocarcinoma: a multicenter comparative study. Ann Surg 2011;254(5):684–93 [discussion: 693].

17. Becker K, Mueller JD, Schulmacher C, et al. Histomorphology and grading of regression in gastric carcinoma treated with neoadjuvant chemotherapy. Cancer 2003;98(7):1521–30.

18. Alderson D, Langley RE, Nankivell MG. Neoadjuvant chemotherapy for resectable oesophageal and junctional adenocarcinoma: results from the UK Medical Research Council randomised OEO5 trial (ISRCTN 01852072). J Clin Oncol 2015;33(Suppl) [abstract 4002].

19. van Hagen P, Hulshof MC, van Lanschot JJ, et al. Preoperative chemoradiotherapy for esophageal or junctional cancer. N Engl J Med 2012;366(22):2074–84.

20. Mariette C, Dahan L, Mornex F, et al. Surgery alone versus chemoradiotherapy followed by surgery for stage I and II esophageal cancer: final analysis of randomized controlled phase III trial FFCD 9901. J Clin Oncol 2014;32(23):2416–22.

21. Stahl M, Walz MK, Stuschke M, et al. Phase III comparison of preoperative chemotherapy compared with chemoradiotherapy in patients with locally advanced adenocarcinoma of the esophagogastric junction. J Clin Oncol 2009;27(6):851–6.

22. Sakuramoto S, Sasako M, Yamaguchi T, et al. Adjuvant chemotherapy for gastric cancer with S-1, an oral fluoropyrimidine. N Engl J Med 2007;357(18):1810–20.

23. De Vita F, Giuliani F, Orditura M, et al. Adjuvant chemotherapy with epirubicin, leucovorin, 5-fluorouracil and etoposide regimen in resected gastric cancer patients: a randomized phase III trial by the Gruppo Oncologico Italia Meridionale (GOIM 9602 Study). Ann Oncol 2007;18(8):1354–8.

24. Cascinu S, Labianca R, Barone C, et al. Adjuvant treatment of high-risk, radically resected gastric cancer patients with 5-fluorouracil, leucovorin, cisplatin, and epidoxorubicin in a randomized controlled trial. J Natl Cancer Inst 2007;99(8):601–7.

25. Nitti D, Wils J, Dos Santos JG, et al. Randomized phase III trials of adjuvant FAMTX or FEMTX compared with surgery alone in resected gastric cancer. A combined analysis of the EORTC GI Group and the ICCG. Ann Oncol 2006;17(2):262–9.

26. Group G, Paoletti X, Oba K, et al. Benefit of adjuvant chemotherapy for resectable gastric cancer: a meta-analysis. JAMA 2010;303(17):1729–37.

27. Macdonald JS, Smalley SR, Benedetti J, et al. Chemoradiotherapy after surgery compared with surgery alone for adenocarcinoma of the stomach or gastroesophageal junction. N Engl J Med 2001;345(10):725–30.

28. Smalley SR, Benedetti JK, Haller DG, et al. Updated analysis of SWOG-directed intergroup study 0116: a phase III trial of adjuvant radiochemotherapy versus observation after curative gastric cancer resection. J Clin Oncol 2012;30(19):2327–33.

29. Lee J, Lim DH, Kim S, et al. Phase III trial comparing capecitabine plus cisplatin versus capecitabine plus cisplatin with concurrent capecitabine radiotherapy in completely resected gastric cancer with D2 lymph node dissection: the ARTIST trial. J Clin Oncol 2012;30(3):268–73.

30. Park SH, Sohn TS, Lee J, et al. Phase III trial to compare adjuvant chemotherapy with capecitabine and cisplatin versus concurrent chemoradiotherapy in gastric

cancer: final report of the adjuvant chemoradiotherapy in stomach tumors trial, including survival and subset analyses. J Clin Oncol 2015;33(28):3130–6.

31. Verheij M, Jansen EPM, Cats A. A multicenter randomized phase iii trial of neoadjuvant chemotherapy followed by surgery and chemotherapy or by surgery and chemoradiotherapy in resectable gastric cancer. J Clin Oncol 2016; 34(Suppl) [abstract: 4000].

32. Schuhmacher C, Gretschel S, Lordick F, et al. Neoadjuvant chemotherapy compared with surgery alone for locally advanced cancer of the stomach and cardia: European Organisation for Research and Treatment of Cancer randomized trial 40954. J Clin Oncol 2010;28(35):5210–8.

33. Lowy AM, Mansfield PF, Leach SD, et al. Response to neoadjuvant chemotherapy best predicts survival after curative resection of gastric cancer. Ann Surg 1999; 229(3):303–8.

34. Lordick F, Ott K, Krause BJ, et al. PET to assess early metabolic response and to guide treatment of adenocarcinoma of the oesophagogastric junction: the MUNICON phase II trial. Lancet Oncol 2007;8(9):797–805.

35. zum Buschenfelde CM, Herrmann K, Schuster T, et al. (18)F-FDG PET-guided salvage neoadjuvant radiochemotherapy of adenocarcinoma of the esophagogastric junction: the MUNICON II trial. J Nucl Med 2011;52(8):1189–96.

36. Bang YJ, Van Cutsem E, Feyereislova A, et al. Trastuzumab in combination with chemotherapy versus chemotherapy alone for treatment of HER2-positive advanced gastric or gastro-oesophageal junction cancer (ToGA): a phase 3, open-label, randomised controlled trial. Lancet 2010;376(9742):687–97.

37. Hofheinz R, Hegewisch-Becker S, Thuss-Patience PC. HER-FLOT: Trastuzumab in combination with FLOT as perioperative treatment for patients with HER2-positive locally advanced esophagogastric adenocarcinoma: A phase II trial of the AIO Gastric Cancer Study Group. J Clin Oncol 2014;32(Suppl):5s [abstract: 4073].

38. Rivera F, Jiménez-Fonseca P, Garcia Alfonso P. NEOHX study: Perioperative treatment with trastuzumab in combination with capecitabine and oxaliplatin (XELOX-T) in patients with HER-2 resectable stomach or esophagogastric junction (EGJ) adenocarcinoma—18 m DFS analysis. J Clin Oncol 2015;33(Suppl 3) [abstract: 107].

39. Fuchs CS, Tomasek J, Yong CJ, et al. Ramucirumab monotherapy for previously treated advanced gastric or gastro-oesophageal junction adenocarcinoma (REGARD): an international, randomised, multicentre, placebo-controlled, phase 3 trial. Lancet 2014;383(9911):31–9.

40. Wilke H, Muro K, Van Cutsem E, et al. Ramucirumab plus paclitaxel versus placebo plus paclitaxel in patients with previously treated advanced gastric or gastro-oesophageal junction adenocarcinoma (RAINBOW): a double-blind, randomised phase 3 trial. Lancet Oncol 2014;15(11):1224–35.

41. Le DT, Uram JN, Wang H, et al. PD-1 blockade in tumors with mismatch-repair deficiency. N Engl J Med 2015;372(26):2509–20.

The Role of Radiotherapy in Localized Esophageal and Gastric Cancer

John Ng, MD[a],*, Percy Lee, MD[b]

KEYWORDS

- Gastrointestinal radiotherapy • Esophageal cancer • Gastric cancer
- Preoperative chemoradiotherapy • Adjuvant therapy • Proton therapy
- MRI radiation therapy

KEY POINTS

- This article reviews the evolving role of radiotherapy in the multidisciplinary management of esophageal, gastroesophageal junction (GEJ), and gastric cancer, summarizing the results of recent clinical trials leading to contemporary accepted treatment approaches.
- A major theme is the evidence supporting the role of radiotherapy in combined modality management, particularly the trend toward its delivery in the neoadjuvant setting.
- The article also reviews novel radiotherapy paradigms and newer radiation technologies such as image-guided radiotherapy and MRI-guided radiotherapy.

INTRODUCTION

Esophageal and gastric cancers remain a major national and global health problem. In the United States, it was estimated that there would be 26,000 new diagnosed gastric cancer cases and 17,000 new cases of esophageal cancers in 2016.[1] For the United States in 2016, gastric cancers were estimated to lead to 10,000 deaths and esophageal cancers to over 15,000 deaths. In China in 2015, the incidence of esophageal and gastric cancers was approximately 478,000 and 679,000 cases, respectively, and the mortality was estimated at 375,000 and 498,000 deaths, respectively.[2] Of particular concern is that in recent decades, the incidence of gastroesophageal junction (GEJ) adenocarcinomas has been increasing. To improve cure rates for these

Disclosure Statements: J. Ng has no conflicts to disclose. P. Lee has a speaking honorarium from Viewray, Incorporated.
[a] Department of Radiation Oncology, Weill Cornell Medical College, New York-Presbyterian Hospital, 525 East 68th Street, N-046, New York, NY 10065, USA; [b] Department of Radiation Oncology, Jonsson Comprehensive Cancer Center, David Geffen School of Medicine, University of California Los Angeles, 200 UCLA Medical Plaza, B265, Los Angeles, CA 90095, USA
* Corresponding author.
E-mail address: Jon9024@med.cornell.edu

Hematol Oncol Clin N Am 31 (2017) 453–468
http://dx.doi.org/10.1016/j.hoc.2017.01.005
0889-8588/17/© 2017 Elsevier Inc. All rights reserved.

hemonc.theclinics.com

patients with poor prognosis, combining chemotherapy, radiotherapy, and surgery in treatment has become a core strategy.

Many strategies of incorporating chemotherapy, radiotherapy, and surgery have been tried over the decades. Using radiation therapy as a way of shrinking tumors or to treat regional disease in esophageal and gastric cancers has an extensive history. In the modern era, radiotherapy has become more refined both in its indications and in its delivery. For example, improved accuracy of delivery has allowed radiation oncologists to treat the gross tumor with smaller margins, sparing normal tissue toxicities along the way. The range of therapeutic radiation dosages, radiation fields, and incorporation with systemic therapy are now better understood. With that refinement, there is now considerable evidence supporting radiation's role in multiple settings for treatments of both esophageal and gastric cancer. As radiotherapy techniques become more precise and radiation toxicities lower, the wider therapeutic window in an anatomically sensitive region will hopefully translate to better clinical outcomes.

This article breaks down radiotherapy's roles in several common clinical settings in the management of localized esophageal and gastric cancers. Radiotherapy has moved earlier in the multimodality management sequence of a patient's treatment, and greater emphasis is placed on using technologies to minimize serious adverse effects. This article emphasizes the increasingly important roles of radiotherapy in the neoadjuvant chemoradiation setting before surgery or in the definitive chemoradiation setting with nonsurgical management. Incremental improvements in the various modalities involved in the care of these patients have led to improved survival of patients with localized esophageal and gastric cancer. There remain many opportunities for the radiation oncology community to further improve outcomes in these diseases, which remain high in incidence and mortality.

RADIOTHERAPY IN ESOPHAGEAL CANCER
Neoadjuvant Chemoradiation in Esophageal Cancer

Chemoradiotherapy before surgical resection (eg, neoadjuvant chemoradiation) in locally advanced esophageal cancer, while sound in principle, only recently has gained broad acceptance as a preferred standard of care treatment option. Critiques and limitations of earlier trials limited the acceptance of the neoadjuvant chemoradiation approach, including issues related to sample size, trial design, and antiquated radiation techniques and doses.

In this context, the CROSS study (chemo radiotherapy for oesophageal cancer followed by surgery study) has become the most influential study in the management of locally advanced esophageal cancer in the past decade, due to the unprecedented survival outcome with acceptable toxicity for patients enrolled in the multimodality management arm of the trial.[3] The CROSS study was a large phase III trial of 366 patients that compared neoadjuvant chemoradiation (41.4 Gy concurrent with weekly carboplatin/paclitaxel) followed by surgery versus surgical resection alone. The results of the CROSS study showed a remarkable median overall survival (OS) of 49.4 months for patients who received neoadjuvant chemoradiation followed by surgical resection versus 24.0 months for those patients who received surgery alone.[4] Toxicities were also reasonable, with less than 20% grade 3 or worse toxicity in the combined modality arm. The results of the neoadjuvant chemoradiation arm in the CROSS study were impressive, not only in demonstrating a marked improvement in local control of the disease, but a significant improvement in negative margin resection rates (92% vs 67%, $P<.001$) and all patterns of recurrence.[5] Local regional control, distant metastatic control, and overall survival outcomes were all on a scale that has now changed standard practice globally. Notably, the pathologic complete response rate in the trimodality arm was 29%. However, in patients with squamous cell histology, the pathologic complete response rate was 49% (18 of 37 patients) compared with 23% (28 of 121 patients) in patients with adenocarcinoma histology. In each arm, 23% of the patients had squamous cell histology. These results suggest that, with the right imaging or blood biomarkers for selecting a favorable response, perhaps half of the patient population with esophageal cancer with squamous cell histology would not require surgery after chemoradiotherapy. Such an approach would further limit the overall treatment morbidity in this subset of the patient population.

Neoadjuvant chemoradiotherapy preceding surgery to improve outcomes was not a newly proposed concept before the CROSS study. Two decades ago, the Dublin Trial had explored the role of neoadjuvant chemoradiation in a prospective, randomized trial randomizing 118 patients with combined chemoradiotherapy (CRT) and surgery compared with surgery alone.[6] The patients on the chemoradiation arm received cisplatin/5-fluorouracil (5-FU) concurrently with esophageal radiotherapy to 40 Gy. The results showed a survival benefit from combined modality arm with a median survival of 16 months, but the poor outcomes of the surgical control group (median OS of 11 months) were raised as a critique of this study. This provocative ground-breaking trial hinted that neoadjuvant chemoradiation may be a superior approach, but it was not convincing enough to those who still favored a surgical approach alone.

Given the results of the Dublin study, the Cancer and Leukemia Group B (CALGB) launched the CALGB 9781 trial.[7] CALGB 9781 differed from the Dublin study in that this phase III study utilized a higher dose of radiation (50.4 Gy with cisplatin and 5-FU), and it had planned to randomize a larger population of patients to receive chemoradiation followed by surgery versus surgery alone. Like the Dublin study, CALGB 9781 also showed a survival benefit with the combined modality approach. After a median patient follow-up of 6 years, overall survival was significantly better in the preoperative chemoradiotherapy cohort over the surgery-alone cohort (5 year OS of 39% vs 16%, P<.008). Furthermore, the rate of complete pathologic response was an unprecedented 40%. Yet skeptics noted that the trial did not accrue many patients—56 patients of a planned 500 patient target accrual—and the conclusions were challenged because of the trial's small patient sample size. It is important to note that a statistically significant improvement in survival was found despite CALGB 9781 being an underpowered study.

Given the limitations and critiques of the Dublin study and the CALGB 9781 study, neoadjuvant treatment remained a contested concept. A meta-analysis comparing neoadjuvant chemoradiation with surgery alone in esophageal cancer also affirmed superiority of the combined modality approach.[8] This meta-analysis reviewed 12 trials and over 1800 patients and favored neoadjuvant chemoradiotherapy with a hazard ratio (HR) of 0.78 (95% confidence interval (CI), 0.70–0.88 I, $P = .001$). Combined with the later impressive results of the CROSS trial, many of the critiques of the earlier trials may have been addressed, and the recent clinical studies support neoadjuvant chemoradiation as an optimal treatment strategy in this disease.

There were several notable findings from CROSS that will influence radiation oncology management and serve as important benchmarks. The radiation dose delivered, 41.4 Gy in 23 fractions, is lower than traditional doses of 45 to 50 Gy or higher. In the setting of concurrent carboplatin/taxol chemotherapy, it has been suggested that radiation doses necessary to sterilize microscopic disease in the primary site may be lower than previous assumptions. This reduced dose may potentially reduce the risk associated with subsequent surgical resection (a similar 4% in-hospital mortality rate for both arms), a widely cited concern with neoadjuvant chemoradiation. There are institutional divides with regards to the radiation dose currently utilized for neoadjuvant chemoradiation in esophageal cancer, and doses ranging from 41.4 Gy to 45 Gy to 50 Gy are currently accepted.[9,10]

One commonly raised issue is that while the CROSS study establishes neoadjuvant chemoradiation as a standard treatment approach, it has not been established whether chemoradiation is superior to chemotherapy alone as the neoadjuvant approach. The German preoperative chemotherapy or radiochemotherapy in esophago-gastric adenocarcinoma trial (POET) provides some insight into these comparative approaches.[11] Like CALGB 9781, the trial did not meet its accrual target, accruing only 119 patients of a target accrual of 354 patients. Yet this underpowered study did note a trend toward improved 3-year survival for the neoadjuvant chemoradiation arm, with a 3-year OS rate of 47.4% versus 27.7% ($P = .07$) and improved median overall survival (33.1 months vs 21.1 months) over neoadjuvant chemotherapy followed by resection. Furthermore, the pathologic complete response rate was higher with neoadjuvant chemoradiation over neoadjuvant chemotherapy (16% vs 2%). The results of these key trials are summarized in **Table 1**. While the POET trial was underpowered, the difference in clinical outcomes would suggest that neoadjuvant chemoradiation should remain the favored strategy moving forward.

DEFINITIVE CHEMORADIATION IN ESOPHAGEAL CANCER

Surgical resection remains a central treatment modality for patients with localized esophageal cancer and provides potentially curative treatment. However, there is now significant clinical evidence that definitive chemoradiation is quite effective in esophageal cancer. The landmark RTOG (radiation therapy oncology group) 0851 trial compared dose-escalated radiation versus chemoradiation, with the latter arm showing a superior 5 year OS rate of 26% versus 0%.[12] Most importantly, long-term survivors were noted with localized esophageal cancer patients in RTOG 0851, showing that chemoradiation potentially could be a curative option.

After RTOG 8501 established chemoradiation as a definitive treatment option, the Intergroup 0123 trial examined whether radiation dose escalation could improve outcomes in localized esophageal patients.[13] The 2 arms of the study tested 50.4 Gy versus 64.8 Gy given concurrently with cisplatin/5-FU. The results of this trial were somewhat unexpected as there were a high number of early deaths in the higher dose arm. It is important to note that in intergroup- 0123, many of the deaths in the high-dose arm occurred prior to the lower dose of 50.4 Gy. Retrospective review of this trial has raised the issue of uneven distribution of patients with significant comorbidities, as these patients did not die of esophageal cancer but of cardiac and pulmonary disease. Regardless of interpretation, the dose-escalated arm in this trial did worse (median OS of 18 months vs 13 months).

Several clinical trials have tried to compare definitive chemoradiation versus chemoradiation followed by surgical resection, particularly in the squamous cell carcinoma population, without clear answers. The results of the German Esophageal Cancer Study Group, the GOCSG trial of 172 patients, showed no significant difference in median overall survival in chemoradiation versus chemoradiation with surgery (median OS of 14.9 months vs 16.4 months respectively, nonsignificant P value [NS]).[14] The results of the French FFCD 9102 study of 444 patients also showed similar survival (median OS of 19.3 months for chemoradiation vs 17.7 months for chemoradiation and surgery, P = NS).[15] Along with the results of the CROSS study, the results from the GOCSG trial

Table 1
The results of key trials for neoadjuvant chemoradiation as a treatment approach in esophageal cancer

Trial	Reference	Comparative Arms	Number of Patients	pCR Rates	Outcome
The CROSS study	van Hagen et al,[3] 2012; Shapiro et al,[4] 2015	Neoadjuvant CRT + surgery vs surgery alone	366	29% (neoadjuvant CRT)	Median OS: 49.4 mo (neoadjuvant CRT) vs 24 mo (surgery)
The Dublin study	Walsh et al,[6] 1996	Neoadjuvant CRT + surgery vs surgery alone	103	25% (neoadjuvant CRT)	Median OS: 16 mo (neoadjuvant CRT) vs 11 mo (surgery)
CALGB 9781	Tepper et al,[7] 2008	Neoadjuvant CRT + surgery vs surgery alone	56	40% (neoadjuvant CRT)	Median OS: 54 mo (neoadjuvant CRT) vs 21.6 mo (surgery)
The POET study	Stahl et al,[11] 2009	Neoadjuvant CRT + surgery vs neoadjuvant chemotherapy + surgery	119	16% (neoadjuvant CRT) vs 2% (neoadjuvant chemotherapy)	Median OS: 33.1 mo (neoadjuvant CRT) vs 21.1 mo (neoadjuvant chemotherapy)

and the FFCD 9102 study would suggest that definitive chemoradiation may be a reasonable standard treatment option for localized esophageal cancer with squamous cell histology.

To further test the definitive chemoradiation strategy, a recent phase II study, RTOG 0246, tested a selective surgical salvage resection strategy after a definitive chemoradiotherapy approach. The study showed that selective salvage surgery was feasible with 23 of the 43 patients able to receive chemoradiation without salvage surgery and a 1-year-overall survival of 71%.[16] A large retrospective multicenter study of 848 patients comparing planned esophagectomy versus salvage esophagectomy following chemoradiotherapy found no significant difference in survival or in-hospital mortality.[17] Selective surgery after definitive chemoradiation remains an area of active investigation.

Similar to the uncertainty regarding dose in the neoadjuvant chemoradiotherapy setting, it currently is unclear what radiation dose is needed in the definitive management of localized esophageal cancer. Would dose escalated chemoradiation lead to excessive toxicities as suggested by intergroup-0123, or was that a misleading outlier result of that arm? Doses ranging from 50.4 Gy to 60 Gy for definitive chemoradiotherapy are often utilized in practice.[10,18] Would modern radiotherapy technologies, such as intensity-modulated radiation therapy (IMRT), enable dose escalation where it would have been excessively toxic with older technologies? Potential of widening the therapeutic window with newer radiotherapy technologies, including IMRT, image-guided radiotherapy (IGRT), particle therapy, and MRI guided therapy will be addressed later in this article.

In conclusion, in the era of improved radiotherapy technologies, definitive chemoradiation may be a reasonable standard treatment option for locally advanced esophageal cancer patients, particularly for those with squamous cell carcinoma. Selective surgery after definitive chemoradiation may be a feasible alternative treatment option for situations where it may be preferable to reserve surgery as an elective option. Finally, definitive chemoradiation without surgery may serve as a potential curative option for inoperable patients.

RADIOTHERAPY IN GASTRIC CANCER
Adjuvant Chemoradiation in Gastric Cancer

Surgical resection is the cornerstone of treatment for gastric cancer treatment. Over recent decades with successive clinical trials, the value of multimodality management for improved outcomes in locally advanced disease has become firmly established. The basis behind its rationale is the high rate of nodal metastases and subsequent locoregional relapse with surgical resection alone.[19]

In a seminal work on second-look surgeries after initial curative surgeries, local recurrences or regional lymph node metastases were found in 88% of 107 examined patients.[20] The most common sites of local relapse are in the gastric bed, the gastric remnant, and regional lymph nodes. These findings provided early evidence that surgery alone is inadequate treatment for patients with locally advanced gastric cancer.

Given the known high rate of local failures, clinical investigators asked whether adjuvant therapy after surgery could improve survival. Intergroup 0116 was a landmark phase III trial that randomized patients between surgery alone versus surgery with adjuvant chemoradiation.[21] The trial randomized 556 patients to either observation or chemoradiotherapy after surgical resection, and the chemoradiation arm was 4 months of 5-FU/leucovorin with 45 Gy of radiotherapy. The results of that seminal study changed practice, as the adjuvant chemoradiation arm showed a superior median overall survival of 36 months versus 27 months for surgery alone. Following its publication, surgical resection followed by chemoradiation became a standard of care treatment option widely utilized for treating patients with locally advanced stage gastric cancer.

This survival difference from Intergroup-0116 has remained significant over long-term follow-up. Long-term analysis with greater than 10 year median follow-up results from Intergroup 0116 still show a substantial overall survival advantage to adjuvant chemoradiation.[22] These results showing an overall survival benefit in stage II-IV non-metastatic gastric adenocarcinoma patients when adjuvant chemoradiotherapy was given after surgery have been validated in multiple large analyses using the Surveillance, Epidemiology, and End Results (SEER) database and large literature-based meta-analyses.[23–26]

The other landmark trial that has influenced management of locally advanced gastric cancer patients is the UK Medical Research Council Adjuvant Gastric Infusional Chemotherapy (MAGIC) trial.[27] In the MAGIC trial, 503 patients were randomized to either surgery alone versus surgery with perioperative chemotherapy. The chemotherapy used was 3 cycles of epirubicin, cisplatin, and 5-FU (ECF) before surgery, followed by 3 cycles of ECF after surgery. This study also showed superior outcomes to a combined treatment approach, favoring the perioperative chemotherapy arm with a 36% 5-year survival rate versus 23% 5 year survival rate for surgery alone. With the results of the MAGIC trial, perioperative chemotherapy also became a widely utilized treatment strategy.

Given the long-term results of the Intergroup 0116 trial and the results of the MAGIC trial, the adjuvant chemoradiation approach and the perioperative approach have become the 2 most common approaches taken toward localized gastric cancer. To date, it is not apparent whether adjuvant chemoradiotherapy with the Intergroup 0116 trial or perioperative chemotherapy through the MAGIC trial should be the preferred strategy in the management of locally advanced gastric cancer patients. What is evident is that some form of combined-modality treatment rather than surgical resection alone is best for this high-risk population.

The optimal adjuvant strategy after surgical resection has also become blurred with more recent studies. The Adjuvant Chemoradiation Therapy in Stomach Cancer (ARTIST) trial randomized 458 patients to either adjuvant chemotherapy (capecitabine/cisplatin) versus adjuvant chemotherapy followed by adjuvant capecitabine-based chemoradiation.[28,29] From that trial, the addition of adjuvant chemoradiation to adjuvant capecitabine/cisplatin chemotherapy did not statistically significantly improve survival. However, the node-positive subgroup did appear to gain a disease-free survival advantage ($P<.05$), leading to the currently accruing ARTIST-II trial, which will test the same strategies in node-positive gastric cancer populations.

Within the past year, investigators from another important phase III study, the Chemoradiotherapy After Induction Chemotherapy of Cancer in the Stomach (CRITICS) trial, have reported their unpublished results.[30] The CRITICS study randomized 788 patients to either perioperative chemotherapy (epirubicin, cisplatin, and capecitabine) versus preoperative chemotherapy followed by adjuvant cisplatin/capecitabine-based chemoradiation. With 4.2 years of median follow-up, there was no statistical difference in overall survival between the 2 arms, 3.5 years (perioperative chemo) versus 3.3 years (pre-operative chemo with adjuvant chemoradiation).[31] Of note, only 47% and 52% of patients were able to complete the perioperative chemotherapy and chemoradiotherapy arms, respectively, putting the spotlight again on the importance of improving the tolerability of the multimodality strategy.

The limited percentage of enrolled patients who were able to complete the intended treatment strategies in CRITICS could potentially affect the interpretation of this unpublished study. Nonetheless, the early reported results suggest that postoperative chemoradiation following preoperative chemotherapy and surgery would require better patient selection to demonstrate potential benefit. The population in whom this aggressive approach may be warranted would be those patients who can tolerate more aggressive therapy and those patients who can be predicted to have a greater likelihood of responding to adjuvant chemoradiation. It has been shown in several phase II trials that response to neoadjuvant chemotherapy predicts for survival.[32] The tailoring of response to treatment strategy is the key concept being tested in a currently accruing national clinical trial, Alliance A021302.[33] The Alliance trial will use early fluorodeoxyglucose positron emission tomography (FDG- PET) treatment response to preoperative chemotherapy to direct further treatment, including potentially resection and adjuvant chemoradiotherapy for nonresponders. The results of this important trial may lead toward a more tailored approach to multimodality gastric cancer management.

NEOADJUVANT CHEMORADIATION IN GASTRIC CANCER

One of the most valuable insights gained from the Intergroup 0116 study, the MAGIC study, the ARTIST trial, and the CRITICS study is that it is challenging to get patients to complete aggressive multimodality treatment for gastric cancer, whether through perioperative strategies or through adjuvant strategies. The goal of improving tolerability of combined treatment and other potential advantages has led to the more recent focus on investigating neoadjuvant chemoradiotherapy as a treatment strategy in locally advanced gastric cancer.

The preoperative chemoradiation approach has been tested in 2 phase II studies, both of which have showed impressive rates of pathologic complete response (pCR) greater than 20% and reasonable tolerability.[34,35] The ability to downstage tumors, with significant numbers of pCR responders, and to improve negative margin resections are 2 of the main confirmed advantages of the neoadjuvant treatment strategy. There are several other potential additional advantages to this approach, including better tolerability of the chemoradiation and a limitation of the perioperative and adjuvant strategies. By administering the chemoradiation before surgery, one may be able to reduce the treatment fields or radiation doses, as demonstrated by the CROSS study for esophageal and GEJ cancers. The target is usually better defined, and the irradiated region has not been surgically affected. The neoadjuvant approach may lead to fewer delays to administration as often occurs for adjuvant strategies. Finally, neoadjuvant chemoradiation may enable clinicians to better biologically stratify and risk stratify locally advanced gastric cancer patients according to treatment response, an advantage that should become even more important in the emerging personalized medicine era.

The potential advantages of neoadjuvant chemoradiation in gastric cancer treatment has led to great interest in a currently accruing, potentially practice-changing, international phase III trial. The Trial of Preoperative Therapy for Gastric and Esophagogastric Junction Adenocarcinoma (TOPGEAR) is a randomized phase III trial led by multiple collaborative groups, which will test perioperative epirubicin/cisplatin/fluorouracil (ECF) chemotherapy versus the experimental arm of preoperative chemoradiation plus perioperative ECF chemotherapy.[36] The TOPGEAR study plans to accrue 752 patients with a primary endpoint of overall survival to investigate whether bringing the chemoradiation approach into the preoperative setting can improve outcomes. There is great excitement, influenced by the CROSS study and others, that the neoadjuvant chemoradiation approach may lead to the optimal

Table 2
Summary of key recent gastric cancer trials

Trial	Reference	Comparative Arms	Number of Patients	Most Common Nonhematologic Toxicities	Outcome
Intergroup 0116	MacDonald et al,[21] 2001; Smalley et al,[22] 2012	Surgery + adjuvant CRT vs surgery alone	556	Gastrointestinal 33%, influenza-like 9%, infection: 6%	Median OS: 36 mo (adjuvant CRT) vs 27 mo (surgery)
MAGIC	Cunningham et al,[27] 2006	Perioperative chemotherapy + surgery vs surgery alone	503	Nausea: 12.3%, vomiting: 10.1%, stomatitis: 4.3%	5 y OS: 36.3% (perioperative chemotherapy) vs 23.0% (surgery)
ARTIST	Lee et al,[28] 2012	Surgery + adjuvant chemotherapy vs surgery + adjuvant chemotherapy + adjuvant CRT	458	Nausea: 12.3%, vomiting: 3.1%, hand–foot syndrome: 3.1%	5 y OS: 75% (adjuvant chemotherapy + adjuvant CRT) vs 73% (adjuvant chemotherapy)
CRITICS Study	Dikken et al,[29] 2011; Verheij et al,[31] 2016	Perioperative chemotherapy + surgery vs neoadjuvant chemotherapy + surgery + adjuvant CRT	788	Not yet reported	Median OS: 3.5 y (Perioperative Chemo therapy) vs 3.3 y (neoadjuvant chemotherapy with adjuvant CRT)
Alliance 021302	Shah et al[33]	FDG-PET nonresponders: surgery + adjuvant CRT vs surgery + salvage chemotherapy	162 (planned)	Not applicable	Not applicable
TOPGEAR	Leong et al,[36] 2015	Perioperative chemotherapy + surgery vs neoadjuvant CRT + perioperative chemotherapy + surgery	752 (planned)	Not applicable	Not applicable

framework for delivering combined modality treatment for locally advanced gastric cancer patients. The key recent gastric cancer trials, such as TOPGEAR, are summarized in **Table 2**.

EMERGING RADIATION TECHNOLOGIES: IMAGE-GUIDED RADIATION THERAPY, PROTON THERAPY, AND MRI-GUIDED RADIATION THERAPY

The promise of the combined modality treatment platform has always been juxtaposed by the concerns of the additive toxicity effects from each additional treatment modality. In neoadjuvant chemoradiation, the particular concern is that preoperative treatment increases the difficulty of an already challenging surgical resection and subsequent recovery.[37] These concerns have been borne out in earlier trials testing combined modality treatments, where combined modality treatments usually led to additional toxicities.[38,39] For example, in the recently presented CRITICS study, only half of enrolled patients were able to complete their treatments as planned, whether it be with perioperative chemotherapy or preoperative chemotherapy followed by adjuvant chemoradiotherapy. It should be a vital aim of ever improving radiotherapy technologies to decrease potential toxicities, either by increasing precision in target delivery or by enabling better avoidance of nearby normal tissue damage.

In esophageal and gastric cancer radiotherapy, it is particularly challenging to deliver radiation within an acceptable therapeutic window. It is difficult to get substantial radiation dose to the esophagus and stomach without excessive radiation doses to the heart, lungs, kidneys, and the spinal cord. Older radiation delivery techniques included delivery with a cobalt-60 system or fluoroscopy-based 2-dimensional radiation delivery systems. Not surprisingly, toxicities were substantial, and escalating radiation doses was extremely difficult during that era. The modern era has brought the advent of computed tomography (CT)-based treatment planning and 3-dimensional conformal radiotherapy techniques, now widely available and commonly utilized radiotherapy techniques in the community.

Even with modern radiotherapy techniques, it is apparent that toxicities are substantial and can affect survival when radiotherapy is delivered in the thoracic and abdominal regions. In the recently published dose escalation lung cancer clinical trial, RTOG 0617, dose-escalated chemoradiotherapy led to worse overall survival, possibly because of excessive cardiac and pulmonary toxicities.[40,41] Radiation oncologists are increasingly using IMRT, a technology based on computer-based inverse treatment planning and other dosimetric advantages compared with 3-dimensional conformal techniques, in the quest for better target coverage and less normal tissue dosage in these regions. IMRT consistently has been demonstrated to offer superior dosimetry in the esophageal and gastric regions, including less cardiac and lung radiation doses.[42–44] For esophageal cancer patients, this improved.

Dosimetry with IMRT has led to a large retrospective analysis demonstrating clinically better outcomes in noncancer-related deaths, locoregional control, and overall survival.[45]

Radiotherapy technologies have moved forward beyond the IMRT era. IGRT perhaps now has become a standard radiotherapy platform for treating esophageal and gastric cancer patients. The presence of a cone beam CT (CBCT) scanner enables image acquisition of the treated region and greater accuracy of the radiation to the specified region. Fiducial markers placed before treatment planning may also help with target delineation and organ motion. Volumetric arc-based therapy (VMAT), generally available in high-volume radiation oncology centers, potentially offers even greater dosimetric advantages relative to IMRT.[46,47]

The latest advances in the radiation technology frontier are the emergence of particle therapy and of MRI-guided radiotherapy. Proton therapy is a technology that has been used for decades to treat various solid malignancies. Its main advantage is the sharper radiation dose fall-off and less integral radiation dose compared with photon irradiation. The recent emergence of proton centers, potentially more than 20 centers in the United States, and the implementation of more precise proton delivery

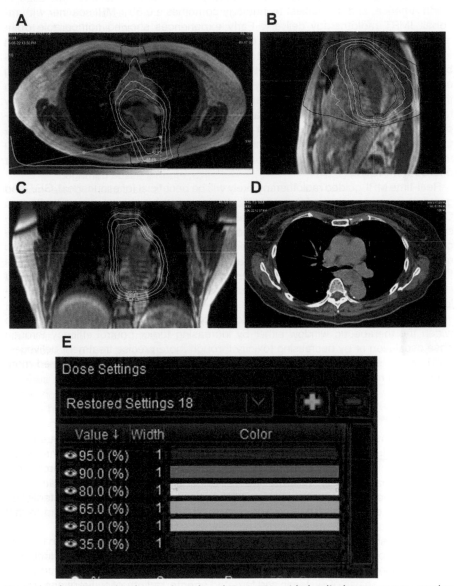

Fig. 1. (A–E) An example of an on-board, real-time MRI-guided radiotherapy treatment plan for a patient undergoing treatment for a locally advanced mid-esophageal carcinoma. (A) An axial plane view of the MRI-guided radiation treatment plan. (B) A sagittal plane view. (C) A coronal plane view. (D) An axial plane view of the same plan based on the CT simulation image. (E) The legend corresponding to the isodose lines in A–C.

techniques have brought renewed interest in utilizing particle radiotherapy in esophageal and gastric cancers. Early clinical studies on proton radiotherapy in esophageal cancer patients have shown encouraging results for this application.[48,49] Further down the horizon is the potential for even greater precision with heavier particles such as carbon ion radiotherapy.

On the imaged-guided radiation delivery front, there has been interest in using on-board, real-time MRI-guided radiotherapy. This technology was first used in North America, and the earliest technology combines a 0.35 T MRI scanner with tricobalt IMRT radiotherapy delivery. Early experiences showed comparable dosimetric comparisons among various disease sites between an MRI-guided system and state-of-the art linear accelerators.[50,51] The added advantage of MRI allows better soft tissue definition for target delineation, better soft tissue contrast during on-board image-guided radiotherapy, tumor tracking in real time using Cine MRI in the sagittal plane, and real-time adaptive radiotherapy. These versatile tools allow radiation oncologists to alter the treatment plan to customize to the patient's anatomy on a given day, while the patient is on the treatment table prior to therapy. MRI-guided technologies offer the promise of intrafractional imaging during radiation treatments in addition to the current capabilities of interfractional imaging currently offered from IGRT.

Real-time MRI-guided radiotherapy likely will be beneficial for esophageal, GEJ, and gastric tumors due to the inherent difficulty in visualizing the disease with CT and CBCT, tumor motion issues related to respiration and cardiac motion, and the radiosensitivity of the neighboring critical structures.[52] **Fig. 1** shows a midesophageal cancer radiotherapy treatment plan created with an on-board, real-time MRI-guided radiotherapy system. The MRI-based plan shows the ability to more precisely define the tumor and the nearby anatomy. There is ongoing work to implement a high-field (1.5 T) MRI on-board with a linear accelerator, although such a system may not be clinically available until 2018 or beyond.

Ultimately, these radiotherapy technologies offer radiation oncologists the ability to widen the therapeutic window either by increasing tumor control efficacy through dose escalation or by decreasing toxicity through more precise treatment deliveries. IMRT, IGRT, particle therapy, and MRI-guided radiotherapy will all be utilized more frequently in radiation treatment centers in the future.

SUMMARY

The management and outcomes of esophageal, GEJ, and gastric cancers are better now than a decade ago. Radiation oncology has become more optimally integrated within the multimodality framework that has emerged in these sites and throughout gastrointestinal oncology. Whereas the role of neoadjuvant or adjuvant treatment in locally advanced disease was once doubted, recent clinical trials have established that they are essential for optimal outcomes. Radiation therapy serves an important role in these contexts.

Concerns are frequently raised about increased toxicities associated with utilizing radiation in combined modality treatments. This therapeutic window may widen with administration earlier in the treatment setting and better patient selection. Current trials will refine use use of systemic and targeted agents, radiotherapy fields and doses, and advancing technologies. Modern and upcoming radiotherapy technologies include image guidance, particle therapy, and MRI-guided radiotherapy, all of which show promise in allowing better soft tissue delineation, more precise radiation delivery, tumor tracking and gating during radiotherapy to spare normal tissue, and real-time adaptive radiotherapy to minimize doses to critical structures due to daily anatomic changes.

Radiotherapy given in the neoadjuvant setting or definitive setting can optimize outcomes. Throughout the gastrointestinal sites, there appears to be a common theme; combined modality treatment before surgery allows for tumor downstaging, better toxicity profiles, and overall better clinical outcomes. As technologies improve and one can better biologically profile individual tumors and tailor patient treatments, combined modality treatment will likely remain the cornerstone strategy in the clinical management of esophageal and gastric cancer patients.

REFERENCES

1. Siegel RL, Miller KD, Jemal A. Cancer statistics, 2016. CA Cancer J Clin 2016;66: 7–30.
2. Chen W, Zheng R, Baade PD, et al. Cancer statistics in China, 2015. CA Cancer J Clin 2016;66(2):115–32.
3. van Hagen P, Hulshof MC, van Lanschot JJ, et al. Preoperative chemoradiotherapy for esophageal or junctional cancer. N Engl J Med 2012;366(22):2074–84.
4. Shapiro J, van Lanschot JJ, Hulshof MC, et al. Neoadjuvant chemoradiotherapy plus surgery versus surgery alone for oesophageal or junctional cancer (CROSS): long-term results of a randomised controlled trial. Lancet Oncol 2015;16(9):1090–8.
5. Oppedijk V, van der Gaast A, van Lanschot JJ, et al. Patterns of recurrence after surgery alone versus preoperative chemoradiotherapy and surgery in the CROSS trials. J Clin Oncol 2014;32(5):385–91.
6. Walsh TN, Noonan N, Hollywood D, et al. A comparison of multimodal therapy and surgery for esophageal adenocarcinoma. N Engl J Med 1996;335:462–7.
7. Tepper J, Krasna MJ, Niedzwiecki D, et al. Phase III trial of trimodality therapy with cisplatin, fluorouracil, radiotherapy, and surgery compared with surgery alone for esophageal cancer: CALGB 9781. J Clin Oncol 2008;26(7): 1086–92.
8. Sjoquist KM, Burmeister BH, Smithers BM, et al. Survival after neoadjuvant chemotherapy or chemoradiotherapy for resectable oesophageal carcinoma: an updated meta-analysis. Lancet Oncol 2011;12:681–92.
9. Ku GY, Ilson DH. Long-term survival with salvage surgery for recurrent esophageal adenocarcinoma after chemoradiotherapy. J Clin Oncol 2015;33(33): 3854–7.
10. Putora PM, Bedenne L, Budach W, et al. Oesophageal cancer: exploring controversies overview of experts' opinions of Austria, Germany, France, Netherlands and Switzerland. Radiat Oncol 2015;10:116.
11. Stahl M, Walz MK, Stuschke M, et al. Phase III comparison of preoperative chemotherapy compared with chemoradiotherapy in patients with locally advanced adenocarcinoma of the esophagogastric junction. J Clin Oncol 2009; 27(6):851–6.
12. Cooper JS, Guo MD, Herskovic A, et al. Chemoradiotherapy of locally advanced esophageal cancer: long-term follow-up of a prospective randomized trial (RTOG 85–01). Radiation Therapy Oncology Group. JAMA 1999;281(17):1623–7.
13. Minsky BD, Pajak TF, Ginsberg RJ, et al. INT 0123 (Radiation Therapy Oncology Group 94–05) phase III trial of combined-modality therapy for esophageal cancer: high-dose versus standard-dose radiation therapy. J Clin Oncol 2002; 20(5):1167–74.

14. Bedenne L, Michel P, Bouché O, et al. Chemoradiation followed by surgery compared with chemoradiation alone in squamous cancer of the esophagus: FFCD 9102. J Clin Oncol 2007;25(10):1160–8.

15. Stahl M, Stuschke M, Lehmann N, et al. Chemoradiation with and without surgery in patients with locally advanced squamous cell carcinoma of the esophagus. J Clin Oncol 2005;23(10):2310–7.

16. Swisher SG, Winter KA, Komaki RU, et al. A Phase II study of a paclitaxel-based chemoradiation regimen with selective surgical salvage for resectable locoregionally advanced esophageal cancer: initial reporting of RTOG 0246. Int J Radiat Oncol Biol Phys 2012;82(5):1967–72.

17. Markar S, Gronnier C, Duhamel A, et al. Salvage surgery after chemoradiotherapy in the management of esophageal cancer: is it a viable therapeutic option? J Clin Oncol 2015;33(33):3866–73.

18. Huang SH, Lockwood G, Brierley J, et al. Effect of concurrent high-dose cisplatin chemotherapy and conformal radiotherapy on cervical esophageal cancer survival. Int J Radiat Oncol Biol Phys 2008;71(3):735–40.

19. Maruyama K, Gunven P, Okabayashi K, et al. Lymph node metastases of gastric cancer. General pattern in 1931 patients. Ann Surg 1989;210:596–602.

20. Gunderson LL, Sosin H. Adenocarcinoma of the stomach: areas of failure in a re-operation series (second or symptomatic look) clinicopathologic correlation and implications for adjuvant therapy. Int J Radiat Oncol Biol Phys 1982;8(1):1–11.

21. Macdonald JS, Smalley SR, Benedetti J, et al. Chemoradiotherapy after surgery compared with surgery alone for adenocarcinoma of the stomach or gastro-esophageal junction. N Engl J Med 2001;345:725–30.

22. Smalley SR, Benedetti JK, Haller DG, et al. Updated analysis of SWOG-directed intergroup study 0116: a phase III trial of adjuvant radiochemotherapy versus observation after curative gastric cancer resection. J Clin Oncol 2012;30(19): 2327–33.

23. Fiorica F, Cartei F, Enea M, et al. The impact of radiotherapy on survival in resectable gastric carcinoma: a meta-analysis of literature data. Cancer Treat Rev 2007; 33:729–40.

24. Valentini V, Cellini F, Minsky BD, et al. Survival after radiotherapy in gastric cancer: systematic review and meta-analysis. Radiother Oncol 2009;92:176–83.

25. Seyedin S, Wang PC, Zhang Q, et al. Benefit of adjuvant chemoradiotherapy for gastric adenocarcinoma: a SEER population analysis. Gastrointest Cancer Res 2014 May;7(3–4):82–90.

26. Stessin AM, Sison C, Schwartz A, et al. Does adjuvant radiotherapy benefit patients with diffuse-type gastric cancer? Results from the surveillance, epidemiology, and end results database. Cancer 2014;120(22):3562–8.

27. Cunningham D, Allum WH, Stenning SP, et al. Perioperative chemotherapy versus surgery alone for resectable gastroesophageal cancer. N Engl J Med 2006;355: 11–20.

28. Lee J, Lim do H, Kim S, et al. Phase III trial comparing capecitabine plus cisplatin versus capecitabine plus cisplatin with concurrent capecitabine radiotherapy in completely resected gastric cancer with D2 lymph node dissection: the ARTIST trial. J Clin Oncol 2012;30:268–73.

29. Dikken JL, van Sandick JW, Maurits Swellengrebel HA, et al. Neo-adjuvant chemotherapy followed by surgery and chemotherapy or by surgery and chemoradiotherapy for patients with resectable gastric cancer (CRITICS). BMC Cancer 2011;11:329.

30. Park SH, Sohn TS, Lee J, et al. Phase III trial to compare adjuvant chemotherapy with capecitabine and cisplatin versus concurrent chemoradiotherapy in gastric cancer: final report of the adjuvant chemoradiotherapy in stomach tumors trial, including survival and subset analyses. J Clin Oncol 2015;33(28):3130–6.
31. Verheij M, Jansen E, Cats A, et al. A multicenter randomized phase III trial of neo-adjuvant chemotherapy followed by surgery and chemotherapy or by surgery and chemoradiotherapy in resectable gastric cancer: first results from the CRITICS study. J Clin Oncol 2016;34(suppl) [abstract: 4000].
32. Lowy AM, Mansfield PF, Leach SD, et al. Response to neoadjuvant chemotherapy best predicts survival after curative resection of gastric cancer. Ann Surg 1999 Mar;229(3):303–8.
33. ClinicalTrials.gov Identifier: NCT02485834.
34. Ajani JA, Mansfield PF, Janjan N, et al. Multi-institutional trial of preoperative chemoradiotherapy in patients with potentially resectable gastric carcinoma. J Clin Oncol 2004;22:2774–80.
35. Ajani JA, Winter K, Okawara GS, et al. Phase II trial of preoperative chemoradiation in patients with localized gastric adenocarcinoma (RTOG 9904): quality of combined modality therapy and pathologic response. J Clin Oncol 2006;24: 3953–8.
36. Leong T, Smithers BM, Michael M, et al. TOPGEAR: a randomised phase III trial of perioperative ECF chemotherapy versus preoperative chemoradiation plus peri-operative ECF chemotherapy for resectable gastric cancer (an international, intergroup trial of the AGITG/TROG/EORTC/NCIC CTG). BMC Cancer 2015;15: 532.
37. Robb WB, Messager M, Goere D, et al. Predictive factors of postoperative mortality after junctional and gastric adenocarcinoma resection. JAMA Surg 2013; 148:624–31.
38. Mariette C, Piessen G, Briez N, et al. Oesophago-gastric junction adenocarcinoma: which therapeutic approach? Lancet Oncol 2011;12:296–305.
39. Cohen DJ, Leichman L. Controversies in the treatment of local and locally advanced gastric and esophageal cancers. J Clin Oncol 2015;33(16):1754–9.
40. Bradley JD, Paulus R, Komaki R, et al. Standard-dose versus high-dose conformal radiotherapy with concurrent and consolidation carboplatin plus paclitaxel with or without cetuximab for patients with stage IIIA or IIIB non-small-cell lung cancer (RTOG 0617): a randomised, two-by-two factorial phase 3 study. Lancet Oncol 2015;16(2):187–99.
41. Movsas B, Hu C, Sloan J, et al. Quality of life analysis of a radiation dose-escalation study of patients with non-small-cell lung cancer: a secondary analysis of the radiation therapy oncology group 0617 randomized clinical trial. JAMA Oncol 2016;2(3):359–67.
42. Kole TP, Aghayere O, Kwah J, et al. Comparison of heart and coronary artery doses associated with intensity-modulated radiotherapy versus three-dimensional conformal radiotherapy for distal esophageal cancer. Int J Radiat Oncol Biol Phys 2012;83(5):1580–6.
43. Fenkell L, Kaminsky I, Breen S, et al. Dosimetric comparison of IMRT vs. 3D conformal radiotherapy in the treatment of cancer of the cervical esophagus. Radiother Oncol 2008;89(3):287–91.
44. Lin SH, Wang L, Myles B, et al. Propensity score-based comparison of long-term outcomes with 3-dimensional conformal radiotherapy vs intensity-modulated radiotherapy for esophageal cancer. Int J Radiat Oncol Biol Phys 2012;84(5): 1078–85.

45. Minn AY, Hsu A, La T, et al. Comparison of intensity-modulated radiotherapy and 3- dimensional conformal radiotherapy as adjuvant therapy for gastric cancer. Cancer 2010;116:3943–52.

46. Yin Y, Chen J, Xing L, et al. Applications of IMAT in cervical esophageal cancer radiotherapy: a comparison with fixed-field IMRT in dosimetry and implementation. J Appl Clin Med Phys 2011;12(2):3343.

47. Ma P, Wang X, Xu Y, et al. Applying the technique of volume-modulated arc radiotherapy to upper esophageal carcinoma. J Appl Clin Med Phys 2014;15(3):4732.

48. Lin SH, Komaki R, Liao Z, et al. Proton beam therapy and concurrent chemotherapy for esophageal cancer. Int J Radiat Oncol Biol Phys 2012;83(3):e345–51.

49. Welsh J, Gomez D, Palmer MB, et al. Intensity-modulated proton therapy further reduces normal tissue exposure during definitive therapy for locally advanced distal esophageal tumors: a dosimetric study. Int J Radiat Oncol Biol Phys 2011;81:1336–42.

50. Kishan AU, Cao M, Wang PC, et al. Feasibility of magnetic resonance imaging-guided liver stereotactic body radiation therapy: a comparison between modulated tri-cobalt-60 teletherapy and linear accelerator-based intensity modulated radiation therapy. Pract Radiat Oncol 2015;5(5):330–7.

51. Merna C, Rwigema JC, Cao M, et al. A treatment planning comparison between modulated tri-cobalt-60 teletherapy and linear accelerator-based stereotactic body radiotherapy for central early-stage non-small cell lung cancer. Med Dosim 2016;41(1):87–91.

52. Kishan AU, Lee P. MRI-guided radiotherapy: opening our eyes to the future. Integr Cancer Sci Therap 2016;3. http://dx.doi.org/10.15761/ICST.1000181.

Management of Metastatic Gastric Cancer

Radka Obermannová, MD, PhD[a], Florian Lordick, MD, PhD[b],*

KEYWORDS

- Gastric cancer • Metastases • Chemotherapy • Radiotherapy • Surgery • Doublet
- Triplet • Sequence

KEY POINTS

- In metastatic gastric cancer, chemotherapy is part of the palliative care concept. A platinum compound (cisplatin or oxaliplatin) plus a fluoropyrimidine (fluorouracil [5-FU], capecitabine, or S-1) is the global standard.
- HER2 is the only predictive marker, and HER2 testing of the primary tumor and/or metastases is warranted before initiation of first-line treatment.
- Selected patients can benefit from triplet combinations, but increased side effects must be considered. Comorbidity, concomitant diseases, and prior therapies should be taken into account for selecting the appropriate therapeutic approach.
- Recent data support the routine use of second-line chemotherapy, either as mono chemotherapy or as a combination of ramucirumab and paclitaxel.

INTRODUCTION

According to the EUROCARE-5 study, 4 of 5 patients with gastric cancer in Europe die within the first 5 years after diagnosis.[1] With 42,280 new cases and 26,420 deaths, gastric and esophageal cancers rank among the most deathly malignant diseases in the United States in 2016.[2] The high mortality rate indicates that a majority of patients diagnosed with gastric and esophageal cancer are primarily diagnosed in stage IV or eventually recur with metastases. The management of metastatic disease is an important health problem. From a patient perspective, prolongation of life, symptom control,

Disclosure Statement: R. Obermannová has received lecture and advisory honoraria from Amgen, Roche, Eli Lilly, and Nordic and has received travel support from Amgen, Merck, Bayer, and Roche. F. Lordick has received research support from GSK and Fresenius Biotech; he has received lecture and advisory honoraria from Amgen, Biontech, BMS, Eli Lilly, Ganymed, Merck-Serono, Merck-MSD, Nordic, and Roche; and he has received travel support from Amgen, Bayer, MSD, Roche, and Taiho.
[a] Clinic of Comprehensive Cancer Care, Masaryk Memorial Cancer Institute, Faculty of Medicine, Masaryk University, Žlutý kopec 543/7, Brno 656 53, Czech Republic; [b] University Cancer Center Leipzig (UCCL), University Hospital Leipzig, Liebigstraße 20, Leipzig 04103, Germany
* Corresponding author.
E-mail address: florian.lordick@medizin.uni-leipzig.de

Hematol Oncol Clin N Am 31 (2017) 469–483
http://dx.doi.org/10.1016/j.hoc.2017.01.006
0889-8588/17/© 2017 Elsevier Inc. All rights reserved.

and quality of life matter. From a society perspective, cost-related and resource-related issues also are important.

Data from the Netherlands indicate that the use of palliative chemotherapy increased, from 5% in 1990% to 36% in 2011, with a strong increase in particular after 2006 (P<.0001).[3] Disappointingly, median overall survival for all noncardia gastric cancers remained constant between 15 weeks (95% CI, 11.9–17.7) and 17 weeks (95% CI, 15.0–20.0) (P = .10). Systemic chemotherapy was revealed, however, as an independent positive prognostic factor in this disease and patients who received chemotherapy had a longer survival.

The options for patients with metastatic disease are increasing. In the past 5 years several new drugs were made available based on positive study results, including targeted drugs like trastuzumab for human epidermal growth factor receptor 2 (HER2)-positive gastric cancer and ramucirumab for cancers that progressed on first-line treatment. As a consequence, median survival has improved from approximately 6 months to 7 months in early studies to approximately 11 months to 12 months in modern studies. This can be seen as the beginning of a new era for treatment of patients with metastatic gastric cancer. Classic chemotherapy is still an important backbone of treatment but — with an increasing knowledge about gastric cancer biology — more biologically targeted options are to come in the near future.

TREATMENT GOALS

According to the World Health Organization, "palliative care is an approach that improves the quality of life of patients and their families facing the problems associated with life-threatening illness, through the prevention and relief of suffering by means of early identification and impeccable assessment and treatment of pain and other problems, physical, psychosocial and spiritual."[4] (**Box 1**). In metastatic gastric cancer, chemotherapy can be part of the palliative care concept. Physicians who apply chemotherapy should follow these goals.

Box 1
Definition of palliative care according to the World Health Organization

- Provides relief from pain and other distressing symptoms
- Affirms life and regards dying as a normal process
- Intends neither to hasten or postpone death
- Integrates the psychological and spiritual aspects of patient care
- Offers a support system to help patients live as actively as possible until death
- Offers a support system to help the family cope during patients' illness and in their own bereavement
- Uses a team approach to address the needs of patients and their families, including bereavement counseling, if indicated
- Enhances quality of life and may also positively influence the course of illness
- Is applicable early in the course of illness, in conjunction with other therapies that are intended to prolong life, such as chemotherapy or radiation therapy, and includes those investigations needed to better understand and manage distressing clinical complications

From World Health Organization (WHO). WHO definition of palliative care. Available at: http://www.who.int/cancer/palliative/definition/en/. Accessed July 29, 2016; with permission.

Symptoms associated with gastric cancer and health-related quality of life can be assessed with specific questions and suitable questionnaires. Validated instruments for assessing symptom load and quality of life are the European Organisation for Research and Treatment of Cancer questionnaires (QLQ-C30 und QLQ-STO22) and the Functional Assessment of Cancer Therapy (FACT) questionnaires, including FACT-G (General), FACT-E (Esophageal), and FACT-Ga (Gastric). Common symptoms that are assessed with these specific instruments are displayed in **Box 2**.[5] Quality of life is strongly influenced by symptom load in a disease like gastric cancer.[6] Systemic chemotherapy can lead to better symptom control and may also stabilize or improve quality of life.[7,8]

Moreover, chemotherapy also prolongs survival.[7,8] In many patients, however, the efficacy of chemotherapy is of short duration. Median survival of patients receiving systemic chemotherapy is less than 1 year in the Western hemisphere and a couple months longer in East Asia, especially in Japan.[8] With platinum-fluoropyrimidine–based chemotherapy, which is the standard of care for first-line treatment of metastatic gastric cancer, several side effects need to be considered. But because symptom control is usually much better with chemotherapy than with best supportive care alone, there is a clear overall benefit of chemotherapy. In addition, modern combinations like oxaliplatin and 5-FU are better tolerated than earlier regimens.[6,8]

In patients older than 65 years to 70 years, an increasing prevalence of comorbidities and impaired organ functions (renal, heart, bone marrow, and so forth) need to be taken into account. Moreover, symptom load and psychosocial needs of older patients are different from those of younger patients.[9] Therefore, overtoxic treatment like docetaxel-containing triplet regimens cannot generally be recommended in older

---

Box 2
Common symptoms in patients with advanced gastric cancer (according to European Organisation for Research and Treatment of Cancer QLQ-C30 and QLQ-STO 22 and Functional Assessment of Cancer Therapy–Gastric)

- Lack of energy
- Fatigue
- Loss of appetite
- Weight loss
- Pain
- Nausea and emesis
- Constipation
- Flatulence and feeling of fullness
- Acid reflux
- Diarrhea
- Dry mouth
- Shortness of breath
- Weak concentration and memory disorder
- Anxiousness and depression

Data from Blazeby JM, Conroy T, Bottomley A, et al. Clinical and psychometric validation of a questionnaire module, the EORTC QLQ-STO 22, to assess quality of life in patients with gastric cancer. Eur J Cancer 2004;40(15):2260–8.

patients with metastatic gastric cancer.[8,10,11] Oxaliplatin and even irinotecan can substitute for cisplatin without compromising the efficacy of chemotherapy.[12]

FIRST-LINE CHEMOTHERAPY

A variety of cytotoxic drugs, including platinum compounds, fluoropyrimidines, taxanes, anthracyclines, and irinotecan, have activity in gastric cancer. With respect to the prolongation of survival, combinations are more effective than monotherapy.[7] A platinum compound (cisplatin or oxaliplatin) plus a fluoropyrimidine (5-FU, capecitabine, or S-1) is the global standard.[8]

Platinum Compounds

For many years, cisplatin was the leading compound to treat patients with gastric cancer.[7] To avoid some of the typical cisplatin-associated side effects, like, for example, nausea and vomiting, renal toxicity, and ototoxicity, other platinum compounds were also investigated. Carboplatin was not sufficiently active in early studies.[13] In contrast, oxaliplatin revealed similar efficacy compared with cisplatin[10,14] if combined with a fluoropyrimidine. The combination of epirubicin/oxaliplatin/capecitabine (EOX) revealed a significant survival benefit compared with epirubicin/cisplatin/5-FU (ECF) (11.2 vs 9.9 months; $P = .02$) in a secondary analysis of the Randomized ECF for Advanced and Locally Advanced Esophagogastric Cancer 2 (REAL-2) study. Compared with cisplatin, neutropenia, alopecia, renal impairment, and thromboembolic events were rarer with oxaliplatin, whereas diarrhea and neuropathy were more common.[14] A smaller randomized trial from Germany confirmed the trend for better efficacy with oxaliplatin compared with cisplatin and an overall more favorable toxicity profile.[10] Patients older than greater than 65 years, especially, had more benefit from oxaliplatin, with a significantly higher tumor response rate, longer progression-free survival, and a trend for better overall survival (13.9 vs 7.2 months; $P = .08$).[10] In summary, oxaliplatin is noninferior to cisplatin with regard to survival and generally better tolerated, with specific advantages in the elderly population.

An alternative to cisplatin-fluoropyrimidine–based chemotherapy is the combination of irinotecan and 5-FU. Irinotecan plus folinic acid and infusional 5-FU (FOLFIRI) showed equal efficacy in 2 randomized studies in comparison with a cisplatin doublet or triplet.[15,16] Quality-of-life analyses from a French study indicate no difference between irinotecan-based and cisplatin-based first-line chemotherapy with regard to the time until deterioration of quality-of-life scores.[16] Thus far, no direct comparison between oxaliplatin-based and irinotecan-based first-line chemotherapy has been published.

Fluoropyrimidines

Two randomized controlled studies investigated the noninferiority of capecitabine compared with 5-FU. The REAL-2 study[14] as well as the ML17032 trial[17] showed that oral capecitabine can substitute for intravenous (IV) 5-FU with regard to efficacy. The markedly increased rate of hand-foot syndrome that was demonstrated in both studies and its potential negative impact on mobility, self-care, and quality of life should be considered when choosing the preferred fluoropyrimidine for an individual patient. On the other hand, replacing IV 5-FU with capecitabine may save hassle and expenses for insertion of a central venous line and potential complications associated with central IV lines, like infection and thrombosis.

Another orally available alternative is S-1, which is a combination of 3 pharmacologic compounds, namely tegafur, gimeracil, and oteracil potassium. Tegafur is a prodrug of 5-FU. S-1 and cisplatin are the most reasonable first-line standards for unresectable advanced gastric cancer in Japan.[8] The application of S-1 for gastric cancer has been delayed, however, in Western countries. One reason for this delay is that the pharmacokinetics of tegafur is affected by polymorphisms in cytochrome P-450 2A6, and consequently 5-FU concentrations in the plasma are more likely to be elevated in patients from Western countries. Therefore, the dose of S-1 was reduced compared with the approved dose in Japan, in the Multicenter Phase III Comparison of Cisplatin/S-1 With Cisplatin/Infusional Fluorouracil in Advanced Gastric or Gastroesophageal Adenocarcinoma Study (FLAGS). FLAGS reported similar survival between S-1 plus cisplatin and infusional 5-FU plus cisplatin arms (8.6 vs 7.9 months; hazard ratio 0.92; 95% CI, 0.80–1.05; $P = 0$ .20). Significant safety advantages were observed in the S-1 plus cisplatin arm, which may be due, at least in part, to the reduced cisplatin dose in the S-1/cisplatin arm.[18] Direct comparison between S-1 and capecitabine in large-scale randomized trials is lacking, but 2 recently published meta-analyses suggest that S-1 is not more effective than capecitabine in the treatment of gastric cancer patients but does exhibit less toxicity with regard to hand-foot syndrome.[19,20] S1 also seems to have a lower cardiovascular toxicity rate. The ongoing Study to Compare Cardiovascular Side Effects of Teysuno Versus Capecitabine (TOFFEE; NCT01845337) is investigating the effect of these 2 drugs on the cardiovascular system.

In summary, the oral 5-FU derivates (capecitabine and S-1) can be combined safely with platinum compounds in patients with advanced gastric cancer and may substitute for IV 5-FU.

Triplet Combinations with Epirubicine or Docetaxel

Combination chemotherapy on the basis of platinum and fluoropyrimidine compounds is a globally accepted standard of care.[8] The benefit of combining 3 cytotoxic drugs (triplet) instead of 2 (doublet) is controversial. The slightly higher efficacy of triplet combinations comes at the price of more toxicity. Side effects may thwart the benefit of triplets compared with doublets.

The additional benefit of anthracyclines is controversial. One meta-analysis reported a survival benefit for the addition of anthracyclines to cisplatin/5-FU (HR 0.77; 95% CI, 0.62–0.95).[21] This analysis was criticized, however, for its few patients (n = 501) and the low validity of the 3 included randomized studies.

In contrast, adding docetaxel to cisplatin and 5-FU was assessed in an adequately powered randomized controlled trial.[22] The phase III TAX 325 study proved the increased efficacy of docetaxel/cisplatin/5-FU (DCF) versus cisplatin/5-FU.[19] The tumor response rate (37% vs 25%), progression-free survival (median 5.6 vs 3.7 months), and overall survival (median 9.2 vs 8.6 months) were significantly better with DCF. The 2-year survival rate was doubled (18.4% vs 8.8%), leading to the approval of docetaxel for first-line treatment of metastatic gastric cancer in North America and Europe. For toxicity reasons, however, it was revealed difficult to implement DCF in clinical practice because the study population of TAX 325 was highly selected, with a median age of 55 years, in whom DCF caused markedly increased hematological and gastrointestinal toxicity. Despite this, quality-of-life analyses showed that the time until definitive deterioration of the global health status compared with baseline was delayed with DCF and patients had a better quality of life.[23]

Modifications of the original DCF protocol were developed. Some investigators changed the scheduling of the 3 drugs[24–26]; others additionally substituted oxaliplatin for cisplatin.[27,28] Modified DCF (IV 5-FU 2000 mg/m^2 for 48 hours; docetaxel 40 mg/m^2 on day 1; cisplatin 40 mg/m^2 on day 3, every 2 weeks) was less toxic than parent DCF, even when supported with growth factors, and was associated with improved efficacy (median overall survival 18.8 vs 12.6 months; $P = .007$). Therefore, modified DCF can be considered a first-line option for selected patients with metastatic gastric or esophagogastric junction adenocarcinoma.[25] Biweekly oxaliplatin in combination with docetaxel and folinic acid/5-FU (two very similar regimens called TEF or FLOT) also displayed a good efficacy with acceptable side effects in phase II studies.[27,28] In patients greater than or equal to 65 years of age, however, FLOT caused greater than 80% grade 3 adverse events and led to significant impairment of quality of life compared with the same chemotherapy without docetaxel.[11]

Direct comparison of anthracycline versus docetaxel-containing triplet regimens in large-scale, randomized controlled trials in metastatic gastric cancer are lacking thus far. Notwithstanding, a total of 553 cases were included in a recently published meta-analysis; 278 received epirubicin-based treatment and 313 received docetaxel. The pooled risk ratio to achieve an objective response and a disease control rate were 1.08 (95% CI, 0.85–1.37; $P = .52$) and 0.90 (95% CI, 0.75–1.08; $P = .27$), respectively. Epirubicin chemotherapy showed a decrease in the risk of neutropenia, anemia, fatigue, asthenia, diarrhea, and neuropathy; docetaxel showed a decrease in the risk of leukopenia, thrombocytopenia, anorexia, nausea and vomiting, stomatitis, and neutropenic fever. The results of this study suggest a comparable activity and efficacy of docetaxel and epirubicin-based chemotherapeutic regimens in metastatic gastric cancer.[29]

In summary, data are not supporting the use of epirubicin or docetaxel-based triplet regimens in all patients with metastatic gastric cancer. Selected patients can benefit from triplet combinations, but increased side effects must be considered. Comorbidity, concomitant diseases and prior therapies should be taken into account for selecting the appropriate therapeutic approach.

First-Line Chemotherapy for HER2-Positive Disease

The Trastuzumab for Gastric Cancer (ToGA) study showed that patients with HER2-positive metastatic gastric and esophagogastric junction adenocarcinoma benefit from the addition of trastuzumab, a monoclonal humanized IgG1 anti–HER2-directed antibody to cisplatin-fluoropyrimidine chemotherapy (median survival 11.1 vs 13.8 months, hazard ratio 0.74; 95% CI, 0.60–0.91; $P = .0046$). Patients for ToGA were selected based on a positive HER2 immunohistochemistry and fluorescence in situ hybridization according to prespecified criteria.[30] The chemotherapy backbone for trastuzumab was capecitabine or 5-FU combined with cisplatin. Meanwhile, data from phase 2 studies and retrospective case-control studies suggest that trastuzumab can be combined safely and effectively with oxaliplatin-fluoropyrimidine combinations.[31–33] Based on ToGA and on the approval status of trastuzumab in many countries, cisplatin-fluoropyrimidine is still the standard chemotherapy backbone but in cases of contraindications against cisplatin, the authors propose combining trastuzumab with an oxaliplatin-fluoropyrimidine doublet.

Unfortunately, lapatinib failed to add the same efficacy as trastuzumab in the TRIO-013/LOGiC trial. A total of 545 patients with HER2-positive advanced gastroesophageal cancer were randomly assigned to receive capecitabine and oxaliplatin (CapeOx) with lapatinib or with placebo. Median overall survival in the lapatinib and placebo arms was 12.2 (95% CI, 10.6–14.2) and 10.5 months (95% CI, 9.0–11.3), respectively, which was not significantly different (hazard ratio, 0.91; 95% CI, 0.73–1.12). Median progression-free survival in the lapatinib and placebo arms was significantly longer, and response rate was significantly higher in the lapatinib arm, 53% (95% CI, 46.4–58.8), compared with 39% (95% CI, 32.9–45.3) in the placebo arm ($P = .0031$).

Preplanned exploratory subgroup analyses showed overall survival in the lapatinib arm was prolonged in Asian and younger patients. In contrast, no correlation was observed between HER2 immunohistochemistry status and survival. In conclusion, the addition of lapatinib to CapeOx did not increase overall in patients with HER2-amplified gastroesophageal adenocarcinoma. There were clear differences in the effect of lapatinib depending on region and age, and future studies could examine this correlation.[34]

Standard Treatment Regimens

Based on scientific evidence and practicability in clinical routine, the authors suggest using 1 of the outlined chemotherapy first-line regimens in patients with metastatic gastric cancer (**Table 1**).

SECOND-LINE CHEMOTHERAPY

Approximately 40% of patients who receive first-line chemotherapy receive second-line chemotherapy on progression.[35] Three randomized studies suggest that second-line monochemotherapy prolongs median overall survival by approximately 1.5 months compared with best supportive care alone.[36–38] Second-line chemotherapy with irinotecan or docetaxel may also improve symptom control and prolong the time until deterioration of quality of life.[36,38] In a phase III study from Japan, paclitaxel showed equal efficacy compared with irinotecan in the second-line setting.[39]

Ramucirumab is a fully human monoclonal IgG1 antibody, which is directed against vascular endothelial growth factor receptor 2 (VEGFR2). Binding of ramucirumab to VEGFR2 antagonizes binding of its activating ligands.[40] In patients with progression on platinum-fluoropyrimidine first-line chemotherapy, the phase III Ramucirumab Monotherapy for Previously Treated Advanced Gastric or Gastro-Oesophageal Junction Adenocarcinoma (REGARD) study showed better median overall survival of 5.2 months in patients in the ramucirumab group compared with 3.8 months in those in the placebo group (hazard ratio 0.776; 95% CI, 0.603–0.998; $P = .047$).[41] Moreover, the phase III Ramucirumab Plus Paclitaxel Versus Placebo Plus Paclitaxel in Patients with Previously Treated Advanced Gastric or Gastro-Esophageal Junction Adenocarcinoma (RAINBOW) showed that overall survival was significantly longer in patients receiving ramucirumab plus weekly paclitaxel than with placebo plus paclitaxel (median 9.6 months [95% CI, 8.5–10.8] vs 7.4 months [95% CI, 6.3–8.4]; hazard ratio 0.807 [95% CI, 0.678–0.962]; $P = .017$).[42] In both studies, quality-of-life parameters were found better with ramucirumab compared with placebo.[41,43]

Currently used chemotherapy regimens for second-line treatment of metastatic gastric cancer are displayed in **Table 2**. Based on scientific evidence and personal experience with the treatment options, the authors recently proposed an algorithm for sequential medical treatment of metastatic gastric cancer[44,45] (**Fig. 1**).

The second-line treatment of patients with HER2-positive gastric cancer is currently not different from treatment of HER2-negative disease. There are no data yet supporting to continue trastuzumab in the second-line setting once they received it in the first line. In addition, the randomized controlled TyTAN phase III study from East Asia and the randomized phase II GastroLap study from Europe failed to show efficacy of lapatinib in the second-line treatment of patients with HER2-positive metastatic gastric cancer.[46,47] Unfortunately, this was also true for trastuzumab emtansine (T-DM1): a recently presented phase II/III study investigating T-DM1, an anti-HER2-directed

Table 1
Recommended first-line treatment regimens investigated in randomized controlled phase II and phase III trials in advanced gastric cancer in North America and Europe

Chemotherapy agents	Dosage (mg/m²)	Application	Response Rate (%)	Median Progression-free Survival (months)	Median Overall Survival (months)
Triplet chemotherapy combinations					
ECX[14]			46.4	6.7	9.9
Epirubicin	50	IV d 1			
Cisplatin	60	IV d 1			
Capecitabine	1250	PO d 1–21			
Q3w					
EOX[14]			47.9	7.0	11.2
Epirubicin	50	IV d 1			
Oxaliplatin	130	IV d 1			
Capecitabine	1250	PO d 1–21			
Q3w					
Modified DCF[25]			49.0	9.7	18.6
Docetaxel	40	IV d 1			
Cisplatin	50	IV d 3			
5-FU	2000	IV d 1 (48 h)			
Q2w					
TEF[28]			46.6	7.7	14.6
Docetaxel	40	IV d 1			
Oxaliplatin	85	IV d 1			
Folinic acid	400	IV d 1			
5-FU	2600	IV d 1 (46 h)			
Q2w					
Doublet chemotherapy combinations					
Cisplatin/capecitabine[17]			46.0	5.6	10.5
Cisplatin	80	IV d 1			
Capecitabine	2000	PO d 1–14			
Q3w					
Western cisplatin + S-1[18]			29.1	4.8	8.6
Cisplatin	75	IV d 1			
S-1	50	PO d 1–21			
Q4w					
FLO (modified FOLFOX)[10]			34.8	5.8	10.7
Oxaliplatin	85	IV d 1			
Folinic acid	200	IV d 1			
5-FU	2600	IV d 1 (24 h)			
Q2w					
FOLFIRI[16]			39.2	5.8	9.7
Irinotecan	180	IV d 1			
Folinic acid	400	IV d 1			
5-FU bolus	400	IV d 1			
5-FU infusion	2400	IV d 1 (46 h)			

(continued on next page)

Table 1
(continued)

Chemotherapy agents	Dosage (mg/m²)	Application	Response Rate (%)	Median Progression-free Survival (months)	Median Overall Survival (months)
Targeted therapy					
Cisplatin/capecitabine/ trastuzumab[30]			46.0	5.6	10.5
Cisplatin	80	IV d 1			
Capecitabine	2000	PO d 1–14			
Trastuzumab cy 1	8 mg/kg	IV d 1			
Trastuzumab>cy1	6 mg/kg	IV d 1			
Q3w					

Abbreviations: cy, cycle; d, day; h, hours; OS, overall survival; PO, per os (by mouth); Q, repeated; w, weekly.

antibody-drug conjugate, also failed to meet its primary endpoint. T-DM1 in second-line HER2-positive gastric cancer did not improve OS compared with taxane standard therapy (8.6 months with taxane vs 7.9 months with T-DM1; hazard ratio 1.15; $P = .8589$).[48]

Table 2
Recommended second-line treatment regimens investigated in randomized controlled phase II and phase III trials in advanced gastric cancer

Chemotherapy agents	Dosage (mg/m²)	Application	Response Rate (%)	Median Progression-free Survival (months)	Median Overall Survival (months)
Monotherapy					
Irinotecan[37]	150	IV d 1	8	NR	6.5
Q2w					
Docetaxel[37]	60	IV d 1	11	NR	5.2
Q3w					
Docetaxel[38]	75	IV d 1	7	3.1	5.2
Q3w					
Paclitaxel[39]	80	IV d 1, 8, 15	20.9	3.6	9.5
Q4w					
Ramucirumab[41]	8 mg/kg	IV d 1	3	2.1	5.2
Q2w					
Combination therapy					
Ramucirumab/paclitaxel[42]			27.9	4.4	9.6
Ramucirumab	8 mg/kg	IV d 1, 15			
Paclitaxel	80	IV d 1, 8, 15			
Q4w					

Abbreviations: d, day; NR, not reported; Q, repeated; w, weekly.

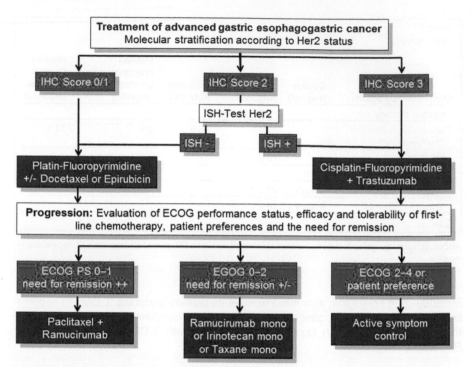

Fig. 1. Proposed treatment algorithm for advanced gastric cancer. ECOG, Eastern Cooperative Oncology Group; IHC, immunohistochemistry; ISH, in situ hybridization. (*Adapted from* Lordick F, Janjigian YY. Clinical impact of tumour biology in the management of gastroesophageal cancer. Nat Rev Clin Oncol 2016;13(6):351; with permission.)

SPECIAL SITUATIONS
Synchronous Metastases

For incurable advanced gastric cancer, palliative resection or bypass surgery is generally indicated in the presence of major symptoms, such as bleeding or obstruction, whereas the usefulness of gastrectomy aimed at reduction of tumor volume in asymptomatic patients was unclear. Findings from previous studies suggested that the addition of gastrectomy to chemotherapy, even in the absence of any serious symptoms, such as bleeding and obstruction, might improve patient survival. Therefore, investigators from Japan and Korea aimed to investigate the superiority of gastrectomy followed by chemotherapy versus chemotherapy alone with respect to overall survival in these patients.[49] The results of the Gastrectomy Plus Chemotherapy Versus Chemotherapy Alone for Advanced Gastric Cancer With a Single Non-Curable Factor (REGATTA) trial were published recently; 175 patients were randomly assigned to chemotherapy alone (86 patients) or gastrectomy followed by chemotherapy (89 patients). After the first interim analysis, the predictive probability of overall survival was significantly higher in the gastrectomy plus chemotherapy group than in the chemotherapy alone group at the final analysis, only 13.2%; so the study was closed on the basis of futility. Overall survival at 2 years for all randomly assigned patients was 31.7% (95% CI, 21.7–42.2) for patients receiving chemotherapy alone compared with 25.1% (16.2–34.9) for those assigned to gastrectomy plus chemotherapy. Because gastrectomy followed by chemotherapy did not show any survival benefit compared with chemotherapy alone in advanced gastric cancer with a single noncurable factor, gastrectomy cannot be justified for treatment of patients with these tumors.[49]

Metastatectomy

Uncontrolled case series suggested prolonged survival for selected patients undergoing hepatectomy, lung metastatectomy, and surgical removal of Krukenberg tumors.[50–52] A recently commenced German trial (RENAISSANCE; NCT02578368) is evaluating whether metastatectomy in conjunction with perioperative chemotherapy could improve outcomes for patients with limited metastatic gastric cancer. Until further evidence is presented, both gastrectomy and metastatectomy should be considered investigational for patients with gastric cancer. The best selection of patients who are good candidates for metastatectomy is still unclear. Response to preoperative chemotherapy and complete resection of a limited number of metastatic sites are favorable prognostic factors.[53]

Peritonectomy

For patients with peritoneal metastases, data from Asian trials support the use of cytoreductive surgery plus hyperthermic intraperitoneal chemotherapy (HIPEC) in selected patients.[54] Randomized data outside of Asia, however, are lacking. A French series demonstrated a median survival of surgery plus HIPEC of 9.2 months, with 5-year survival of 13% for all patients and 23% for those who had complete cytoreductive surgery.[55] Currently, this approach must be considered investigational. Peritonectomy and perioperative chemotherapy plus HIPEC is currently compared with peritonectomy and perioperative chemotherapy in a prospective randomized controlled study run in Germany (GASTRIPEC; EudraCT number: 2006-006088-22).

SUMMARY AND PRACTICAL CONCLUSION

Although the prognosis of metastatic gastric cancer remains limited, a variety of new medical and nonmedical treatment options were implemented in the past decade. Effective sequential treatment, including different treatment lines and combining different treatment modalities, is now, step-by-step, becoming reality in gastric cancer. Science-based treatment elements, like first-line and second-line standard chemotherapy, which should be given to a majority of patients, should be discriminated from non–evidence-based treatment options, which should be critically discussed on a case-by-case basis. An experienced multidisciplinary tumor board should be consulted to develop balanced recommendations for patients with metastatic gastric cancer. For all therapeutic options, potential benefit should be carefully weighed against potential harm in this aggressive disease, which leads to fragility and considerable morbidity.

REFERENCES

1. De Angelis R, Sant M, Coleman MP, et al. Cancer survival in Europe 1999-2007 by country and age: results of EUROCARE–5-a population-based study. Lancet Oncol 2014;15:23–34.
2. Siegel RL, Miller KD, Jemal A. Cancer statistics, 2016. CA Cancer J Clin 2016;66: 7–30.
3. Bernards N, Creemers GJ, Nieuwenhuijzen GA, et al. No improvement in median survival for patients with metastatic gastric cancer despite increased use of chemotherapy. Ann Oncol 2013;24:3056–60.

4. WHO. World Health Organization. Available at: http://www.who.int/cancer/palliative/definition/en/. Accessed 29 July, 2016.

5. Blazeby JM, Conroy T, Bottomley A, et al. Clinical and psychometric validation of a questionnaire module, the EORTC QLQ-STO 22, to assess quality of life in patients with gastric cancer. Eur J Cancer 2004;40:2260–8.

6. Al-Batran SE, Ajani JA. Impact of chemotherapy on quality of life in patients with metastatic esophagogastric cancer. Cancer 2010;116:2511–8.

7. Wagner AD, Unverzagt S, Grothe W, et al. Chemotherapy for advanced gastric cancer. Cochrane Database Syst Rev 2010;(3):CD004064.

8. Lordick F, Lorenzen S, Yamada Y, et al. Optimal chemotherapy for advanced gastric cancer: is there a global consensus? Gastric Cancer 2014;17:213–25.

9. Morita T, Kuriya M, Miyashita M, et al. Symptom burden and achievement of good death of elderly cancer patients. J Palliat Med 2014;17:887–93.

10. Al-Batran SE, Hartmann JT, Probst S, et al. Phase III trial in metastatic gastroesophageal adenocarcinoma with fluorouracil, leucovorin plus either oxaliplatin or cisplatin: a study of the Arbeitsgemeinschaft Internistische Onkologie. J Clin Oncol 2008;26:1435–42.

11. Al-Batran SE, Pauligk C, Homann N, et al. The feasibility of triple-drug chemotherapy combination in older adult patients with oesophagogastric cancer: a randomised trial of the Arbeitsgemeinschaft Internistische Onkologie (FLOT65+). Eur J Cancer 2013;49:835–42.

12. Petrelli F, Zaniboni A, Coinu A, et al. Cisplatin or not in advanced gastric cancer: a systematic review and meta-analysis. PLoS One 2013;8:e83022.

13. Preusser P, Wilke H, Achterrath W, et al. Phase II study of carboplatin in untreated inoperable advanced stomach cancer. Eur J Cancer 1990;26:1108–9.

14. Cunningham D, Starling N, Rao S, et al. Capecitabine and oxaliplatin for advanced esophagogastric cancer. N Engl J Med 2008;358:36–46.

15. Dank M, Zaluski J, Barone C, et al. Randomized phase III study comparing irinotecan combined with 5-fluorouracil and folinic acid to cisplatin combined with 5-fluorouracil in chemotherapy naive patients with advanced adenocarcinoma of the stomach or esophagogastric junction. Ann Oncol 2008;19:1450–7.

16. Guimbaud R, Louvet C, Ries P, et al. Prospective, randomized, multicenter, phase III study of fluorouracil, leucovorin, and irinotecan versus epirubicin, cisplatin, and capecitabine in advanced gastric adenocarcinoma: a French intergroup (Federation Francophone de Cancerologie Digestive, Federation Nationale des Centres de Lutte Contre le Cancer, and Groupe Cooperateur Multidisciplinaire en Oncologie) study. J Clin Oncol 2014;32:3520–6.

17. Kang YK, Kang WK, Shin DB, et al. Capecitabine/cisplatin versus 5-fluorouracil/cisplatin as first-line therapy in patients with advanced gastric cancer: a randomised phase III noninferiority trial. Ann Oncol 2009;20:666–73.

18. Ajani JA, Rodriguez W, Bodoky G, et al. Multicenter phase III comparison of cisplatin/S-1 with cisplatin/infusional fluorouracil in advanced gastric or gastroesophageal adenocarcinoma study: the FLAGS trial. J Clin Oncol 2010;28:1547–53.

19. He MM, Wu WJ, Wang F, et al. S-1-based chemotherapy versus capecitabine-based chemotherapy as first-line treatment for advanced gastric carcinoma: a meta-analysis. PLoS One 2013;8:e82798.

20. He AB, Peng XL, Song J, et al. Efficacy of S-1 vs capecitabine for the treatment of gastric cancer: a meta-analysis. World J Gastroenterol 2015;21:4358–64.

21. Wagner AD, Grothe W, Haerting J, et al. Chemotherapy in advanced gastric cancer: a systematic review and meta-analysis based on aggregate data. J Clin Oncol 2006;24:2903–9.

22. Van Cutsem E, Moiseyenko VM, Tjulandin S, et al. Phase III study of docetaxel and cisplatin plus fluorouracil compared with cisplatin and fluorouracil as first-line therapy for advanced gastric cancer: a report of the V325 Study Group. J Clin Oncol 2006;24:4991–7.

23. Ajani JA, Moiseyenko VM, Tjulandin S, et al. Quality of life with docetaxel plus cisplatin and fluorouracil compared with cisplatin and fluorouracil from a phase III trial for advanced gastric or gastroesophageal adenocarcinoma: the V-325 Study Group. J Clin Oncol 2007;25:3210–6.

24. Lorenzen S, Hentrich M, Haberl C, et al. Split-dose docetaxel, cisplatin and leucovorin/fluorouracil as first-line therapy in advanced gastric cancer and adenocarcinoma of the gastroesophageal junction: results of a phase II trial. Ann Oncol 2007;18:1673–9.

25. Shah MA, Janjigian YY, Stoller R, et al. Randomized multicenter phase ii study of modified docetaxel, cisplatin, and fluorouracil (DCF) versus DCF plus growth factor support in patients with metastatic gastric adenocarcinoma: a study of the us gastric cancer consortium. J Clin Oncol 2015;33:3874–9.

26. Tebbutt NC, Cummins MM, Sourjina T, et al. Randomised, non-comparative phase II study of weekly docetaxel with cisplatin and 5-fluorouracil or with capecitabine in oesophagogastric cancer: the AGITG ATTAX trial. Br J Cancer 2010;102:475–81.

27. Al-Batran SE, Hartmann JT, Hofheinz R, et al. Biweekly fluorouracil, leucovorin, oxaliplatin, and docetaxel (FLOT) for patients with metastatic adenocarcinoma of the stomach or esophagogastric junction: a phase II trial of the Arbeitsgemeinschaft Internistische Onkologie. Ann Oncol 2008;19:1882–7.

28. Van Cutsem E, Boni C, Tabernero J, et al. Docetaxel plus oxaliplatin with or without fluorouracil or capecitabine in metastatic or locally recurrent gastric cancer: a randomized phase II study. Ann Oncol 2015;26:149–56.

29. Petrioli R, Roviello G, Zanotti L, et al. Epirubicin-based compared with docetaxel-based chemotherapy for advanced gastric carcinoma: a systematic review and meta-analysis. Crit Rev Oncol Hematol 2016;102:82–8.

30. Bang YJ, Van Cutsem E, Feyereislova A, et al. Trastuzumab in combination with chemotherapy versus chemotherapy alone for treatment of HER2-positive advanced gastric or gastro-oesophageal junction cancer (ToGA): a phase 3, open-label, randomised controlled trial. Lancet 2010;376:687–97.

31. Ryu MH, Yoo C, Kim JG, et al. Multicenter phase II study of trastuzumab in combination with capecitabine and oxaliplatin for advanced gastric cancer. Eur J Cancer 2015;51:482–8.

32. Soularue É, Cohen R, Tournigand C, et al. Efficacy and safety of trastuzumab in combination with oxaliplatin and fluorouracil-based chemotherapy for patients with HER2-positive metastatic gastric and gastro-oesophageal junction adenocarcinoma patients: a retrospective study. Bull Cancer 2015;102:324–31.

33. Gong J, Liu T, Fan Q, et al. Optimal regimen of trastuzumab in combination with oxaliplatin/capecitabine in first-line treatment of HER2-positive advanced gastric cancer (CGOG1001): a multicenter, phase II trial. BMC Cancer 2016;16:68.

34. Hecht JR, Bang YJ, Qin SK, et al. Lapatinib in combination with capecitabine plus oxaliplatin in human epidermal growth factor receptor 2-positive advanced or metastatic gastric, esophageal, or gastroesophageal adenocarcinoma: TRIO-013/LOGiC–a randomized phase III Trial. J Clin Oncol 2016;34:443–51.

35. Thallinger CM, Raderer M, Hejna M. Esophageal cancer: a critical evaluation of systemic second-line therapy. J Clin Oncol 2011;29:4709–14.

36. Thuss-Patience PC, Kretzschmar A, Bichev D, et al. Survival advantage for irinotecan versus best supportive care as second-line chemotherapy in gastric cancer–a randomised phase III study of the Arbeitsgemeinschaft Internistische Onkologie (AIO). Eur J Cancer 2011;47:2306–14.

37. Kang JH, Lee SI, Lim do H, et al. Salvage chemotherapy for pretreated gastric cancer: a randomized phase III trial comparing chemotherapy plus best supportive care with best supportive care alone. J Clin Oncol 2012;30:1513–8.

38. Ford HE, Marshall A, Bridgewater JA, et al. Docetaxel versus active symptom control for refractory oesophagogastric adenocarcinoma (COUGAR-02): an open-label, phase 3 randomised controlled trial. Lancet Oncol 2014;15:78–86.

39. Hironaka S, Ueda S, Yasui H, et al. Randomized, open-label, phase III study comparing irinotecan with paclitaxel in patients with advanced gastric cancer without severe peritoneal metastasis after failure of prior combination chemotherapy using fluoropyrimidine plus platinum: WJOG 4007 trial. J Clin Oncol 2013;31:4438–44.

40. Jayson GC, Kerbel R, Ellis LM, et al. Antiangiogenic therapy in oncology: current status and future directions. Lancet 2016;388(10043):518–29.

41. Fuchs CS, Tomasek J, Yong CJ, et al. Ramucirumab monotherapy for previously treated advanced gastric or gastro-oesophageal junction adenocarcinoma (REGARD): an international, randomised, multicentre, placebo-controlled, phase 3 trial. Lancet 2014;383:31–9.

42. Wilke H, Muro K, Van Cutsem E, et al. Ramucirumab plus paclitaxel versus placebo plus paclitaxel in patients with previously treated advanced gastric or gastro-oesophageal junction adenocarcinoma (RAINBOW): a double-blind, randomised phase 3 trial. Lancet Oncol 2014;15:1224–35.

43. Al-Batran SE, Van Cutsem E, Oh SC, et al. Quality-of-life and performance status results from the phase III RAINBOW study of ramucirumab plus paclitaxel versus placebo plusvpaclitaxel in patients with previously treated gastric or gastroesophagealvjunction adenocarcinoma. Ann Oncol 2016;27:673–9.

44. Lordick F, Janjigian YY. Clinical impact of tumour biology in the management of gastroesophageal cancer. Nat Rev Clin Oncol 2016;13:348–60.

45. Obermannová R, Lordick F. Insights into next developments in advanced gastric cancer. Curr Opin Oncol 2016;28:367–75.

46. Satoh T, Xu RH, Chung HC, et al. Lapatinib plus paclitaxel versus paclitaxel alone in the second-line treatment of HER2-amplified advanced gastric cancer in Asian populations: TyTAN–a randomized, phase III study. J Clin Oncol 2014;32:2039–49.

47. Lorenzen S, Riera Knorrenschild J, Haag GM, et al. Lapatinib versus lapatinib plus capecitabine as second-line treatment in human epidermal growth factor receptor 2-amplified metastatic gastro-oesophageal cancer: a randomised phase II trial of the Arbeitsgemeinschaft Internistische Onkologie. Eur J Cancer 2015;51:569–76.

48. Kang YK, Shah MA, Ohtsu A, et al. A randomized, open-label, multicenter, adaptive phase 2/3 study of trastuzumab emtansine (T-DM1) versus a taxane (TAX) in patients (pts) with previously treated HER2-positive locally advanced or metastatic gastric/gastroesophageal junction adenocarcinoma (LA/MGC/GEJC). Gastrointestinal Cancer Symposium 2016; abstract 5.

49. Fujitani K, Yang HK, Mizusawa J, et al. Gastrectomy plus chemotherapy versus chemotherapy alone for advanced gastric cancer with a single non-curable factor

(REGATTA): a phase 3, randomised controlled trial. Lancet Oncol 2016;17: 309–18.

50. Markar SR, Mikhail S, Malietzis G, et al. Influence of surgical resection of hepatic metastases from gastric adenocarcinoma on long-term survival: systematic review and pooled analysis. Ann Surg 2016;263:1092–101.

51. Shiono S, Sato T, Horio H, et al. Outcomes and prognostic factors of survival after pulmonary resection for metastatic gastric cancer. Eur J Cardiothorac Surg 2013; 43:e13–6.

52. Rosa F, Marrelli D, Morgagni P, et al. Krukenberg tumors of gastric origin: the rationale of surgical resection and perioperative treatments in a multicenter western experience. World J Surg 2016;40:921–8.

53. Blank S, Lordick F, Dobritz M, et al. A reliable risk score for stage IV esophagogastric cancer. Eur J Surg Oncol 2013;39:823–30.

54. Yang XJ, Huang CQ, Suo T, et al. Cytoreductive surgery and hyperthermic intraperitoneal chemotherapy improves survival of patients with peritoneal carcinomatosis from gastric cancer: final results of a phase III randomized clinical trial. Ann Surg Oncol 2011;18:1575–81.

55. Glehen O, Gilly FN, Arvieux C, et al. Peritoneal carcinomatosis from gastric cancer: a multi-institutional study of 159 patients treated by cytoreductive surgery combined with perioperative intraperitoneal chemotherapy. Ann Surg Oncol 2010;17:2370–7.

Emerging Targeted Therapies

The Evolving Role of Checkpoint Inhibitors in the Management of Gastroesophageal Cancer

Adrian G. Murphy, MB, BCh, PhD, Ronan J. Kelly, MB, BCh, MBA*

KEYWORDS

- Immune checkpoint • Immunotherapy • Programmed death-1
- Cytotoxic T lymphocyte associated protein −4 • Pembrolizumab • Nivolumab

KEY POINTS

- The connection between inflammation and malignancy has long been recognized in gastric and esophageal cancers.
- Given the considerable success of immune checkpoint inhibitors in other tumor types (eg, lung cancer and melanoma), much attention is being paid to furthering their role in gastric and esophageal cancers.
- The Cancer Genome Atlas has provided further details of the molecular heterogeneity of these tumors, which may help predict responsiveness to immune checkpoint inhibitors.
- This article discusses the rationale for investigating these agents in gastroesophageal (GE) cancer and summarizes the relevant clinical trial data and ongoing studies.

INTRODUCTION

The link between chronic inflammation, infection, and malignancy has long been recognized in both esophageal and gastric cancers. For years, it has been postulated that targeting the immune system in upper gastrointestinal (GI) cancers may lead to improved outcomes in tumors that have proved inherently resistant to novel systemic treatments as a result of histologic, molecular, and etiologic heterogeneity. Although first-line therapy responses of 50% to 60% are typical with systemic chemotherapy in metastatic disease, additional efficacy in the second-line and third-line settings has been limited despite the addition of the targeted agents

Commercial and Financial Conflicts of Interest: Dr R.J. Kelly has received grant funding from Bristol-Myers Squibb.
The Sidney Kimmel Comprehensive Cancer Center, Johns Hopkins Medicine, The Bunting Blaustein Cancer Research Building, 1650 Orleans Street, Room G93, Baltimore, MD 21231, USA
* Corresponding author.
E-mail address: rkelly25@jhmi.edu

trastuzumab and ramucirumab.[1,2] Recently, a phase II/III Gatsby study of ado-trastuzumab emtansine (T-DM1) was negative in the second-line setting compared with paclitaxel/docetaxel.[3] This highlights many of the difficulties oncologists have faced in treating upper GI tumors. Continued targeting of HER2 with novel drugs was expected to result in improved overall survival (OS) but it now seems that up to 35% of patients can have down-regulation of initially positive HER2 overexpression/amplification while receiving first-line trastuzumab. This is not a recognized phenomenon in breast cancer, where continued targeting of HER2 is standard of care. In addition, the lack of identifiable common oncogenic driver mutations in upper GI tumors has led to the hope that the use of checkpoint inhibitors, notably programmed death (PD)-1 inhibitors, and future combination studies can lead to substantial benefits, as seen in other common tumors, such as melanoma, non-small cell lung cancer (NSCLC), and renal cell and bladder carcinomas. This article describes the rationale for investigating checkpoint inhibitors in GE cancer, explores some of the current understandings of the immune microenvironment in these diverse tumors, and provides a synopsis of both ongoing studies and the clinical trial data published to date.

RATIONALE FOR INVESTIGATING CHECKPOINT INHIBITORS IN GASTROESOPHAGEAL CANCER

Tumors escape immune surveillance by several mechanisms, of which 4 groups have been proposed on the basis of their programmed death ligand (PD-L)-1 status and the presence or absence of tumor infiltrating lymphocytes (TILs). These include type I (PD-L1[pos] with TILs driving adaptive immune resistance), type II (PD-L1[neg] with no TIL indicating immune ignorance), type III (PD-L1[pos] with no TIL indicating intrinsic resistance), and type IV (PD-L1[neg] with TIL present indicating the role of other suppressor[s] in promoting immune tolerance).[4] The authors have previously reported that in resected gastric cancers, enhanced CD8$^+$ T cell infiltration in tumors and peritumoral interfaces occurs in patients that were also PD-L1$^+$ compared with those who were PD-L$^-$.[5] When CD8$^+$ T-cell densities were categorized into low, mid, and high, 89% of stroma PD-L1$^+$ tumors had high CD8$^+$ densities. This highlights the importance of the linkage between CD8$^+$ T cells, thought to be a source of cytokines, such as IFNγ, and up-regulation of PD-L1 or the so-called adaptive immuneresponse. Additional work is required in GE cancer to understand which patients are more likely to respond to single-agent checkpoint inhibition and which will require combination strategies. In melanoma, extensive work has been done to demonstrate that a high proportion of type I and type II microenvironments are seen[6] and this can explain the high response rates in this tumor type to PD-1 inhibitors. This information has yet to be defined in GE cancers. At present, there is not a clear understanding of what the early events are that leads to the aberrant expression of PD-1/PD-L1 by tumor cells and/or host immune cells. Genomic aberrations in tumor cells that lead to aberrant PD-L1 expression have been proposed and microsatellite instability (MSI) may have a predictive role as may Epstein Barr Virus (EBV) status.[7,8] Emerging data suggest that negative immune checkpoint proteins are usually up-regulated in tumor tissues with a T-cell inflamed phenotype and that infiltration of tumors by effector T cells is necessary to drive up-regulation of immune checkpoints.[9] These findings suggest that targeting the PD-1/PD-L1 axis in GE cancers may only be clinically effective for the subgroup of tumors that contain tumor-infiltrating immune cells. Additional factors that suggest GE cancers may respond to checkpoint inhibition include

- High somatic mutation burden
- Chronic inflammation
- Genomic instability
- Infection

High Somatic Burden

Recent advances in next-generation sequencing have allowed investigators to appreciate the complexity and diversity of the somatic mutations underlying the development of common malignancies.[10] This technology allows deciphering mutational signatures and offers ways to predict responsiveness to immunotherapeutics. Although multiple factors are involved, it is thought that high somatic mutational burden may be important and only melanoma and lung and bladder cancers display a more mutated profile than GE cancers.[10] Continued research on the link between mutation burden and the T-cell inflamed phenotype may be more predictive of response than the number of mutations alone.

Chronic Inflammation

GE cancers develop in part as a result of prolonged chronic gastric reflux (Gastroesophageal Reflux Disease [GERD])–induced inflammation. In response to GERD, the occurrence of Barrett metaplasia is accompanied by a change from an acute (T helper 1 cell) immune response associated with interferon (IFN)-γ expression to a T helper 2 chronic inflammation with production of interleukin (IL)-4/IL-13, which has been reported to result in an immunosuppressive, tumor-promoting microenvironment.[11,12] This suggests that immunotherapeutics may have a significant role to play in earlier-stage disease, and studies investigating both neoadjuvant and adjuvant strategies in stage II/III esophageal cancer are either in development or are accruing. It is possible that future studies may investigate checkpoint inhibitors in stage I or in situ carcinomas but given the excellent results with localized treatment this is not certain.

Genomic Instability

Defective mismatch repair genes (MMRs) have been identified as predictive of response to PD-1 inhibition because somatic mutations have the potential to encode nonself immunogenic neoantigens.[8] Whole-exome sequencing has demonstrated a mean of 1782 somatic mutations in MMR-deficient tumors compared with approximately 73 in MMR-proficient tumors.[8] An immunologic assessment of the immune microenvironment in MMR-deficient tumors has demonstrated strong expression of several immune checkpoint ligands, notably, PD-1/PD-L1, lymphocyte-activation gene 3 (LAG3), indoleamine 2,3-dioxygenase (IDO), and cytotoxic T-lymphocyte associated (CTLA)-4, which help confer resistance to immunologic attack.[13] MMR deficiency has been identified in 17% to 21% of gastric cancers, and preliminary data indicate a higher response rate in these patients of approximately 50%.[14] Ongoing and future studies in GE cancer will likely stratify according to MSI status.

Infection

Recent data from The Cancer Genome Atlas highlighted the EBV subtype (9%) as a potentially promising group to investigate checkpoint inhibitors.[7] EBV-positive gastric cancers occurred predominantly in the gastric fundus or body and were noted more commonly in men. The investigators described a recurrent amplification at 9p24.1, which is the locus containing *JAK2* but also *CD274* and *PDCD1LG2*, which encode PD-L1 and PD-L2, respectively. These 9p amplifications occurred in 15% of

EBV-driven gastric tumors and result in enhanced neoepitope presentation.[7] Ongoing studies are evaluating checkpoint inhibitors in EBV-positive gastric cancer (NCT02488759).

PROGRAMMED DEATH LIGAND 1 EXPRESSION IN ESOPHAGEAL AND GASTRIC CANCER

Several investigators have determined that PD-L1 expression occurs in approximately 40% of gastric and GE junction (GEJ) cancers.[15–17] The recent KEYNOTE-012 phase 1b trial assessed pembrolizumab in patients with PD-L1[+] advanced gastric cancer as determined using the 22C3 antibody staining both tumor cells and mononuclear inflammatory cells. Of the 162 patients screened, 65 (40%) were considered PD-L1[+] tumors. The investigators report that to detect responses in gastric cancer, it was necessary for them to assess PD-L1 expression by immune cells as opposed to tumor cell expression exclusively.[18] The authors previously reported that, of 34 resected gastric or GEJ tumors stained by immunohistochemistry using the 5H1 clone, only 12% of tumors demonstrated cell membranous PD-L1 expression whereas 44% showed expression within the immune stroma.[5] How this has an impact on disease response to single-agent PD-1 inhibition in GE cancer remains to be seen, but this pattern is different from that seen in NSCLC, where more membranous expression is observed.

PREDICTIVE BIOMARKERS TO GUIDE USE OF CHECKPOINT INHIBITORS IN GASTROESOPHAGEAL CANCER
Programmed Death Ligand 1/Programmed Death Ligand 2 Status

Using PD-L1 as a predictive biomarker is controversial for all solid tumors at present, and this remains true for upper GI tumors. Several clinical trials, discussed later, have either preselected or not preselected patients for PD-1/PD-L1 inhibitors based on PD-L1 expression.

KEYNOTE-012 preselected patients for enrollment and only those subjects with PD-L1[+] tumors were considered eligible for the trial. PD-L1 positivity was defined as membrane staining in at least 1% of scorable cells or the presence of a distinctive interface pattern. The problems posed by the numerous assays/antibodies used to assess PD-L1 status are well described. This allied with tumor heterogeneity, reproducibility of results, and no simplified scoring system makes the use of PD-L1 as a predictive biomarker difficult at present in GE cancer. Although responses are higher in PD-L1[+] tumors, there are responses in PD-L1[−] tumors. Unlike in other tumors, there are no data on PD-L2 expression, with moderate/strong epithelial expression occurring in 51.7% of esophageal adenocarcinomas and up to 81.6% reported as having weak expression.[19] This may have implications for the efficacy of PD-L1 inhibitors versus PD-1 inhibitors in GE cancer and may explain in part the lower responses seen in the preliminary data, presented as abstracts with the PD-L1 inhibitors to date. Additionally, there is a question as to why a majority of esophageal cancers can harbor 2 distinct checkpoints and what the implications for this are for future clinical trials.

Mononuclear Inflammatory Score

In addition to PD-L1 staining, a mononuclear inflammatory cell density score of 0 to 4 was also described in KEYNOTE-012.[18] Of the 9 patients who had a score greater than or equal to 3, 4 of 9 (44%) had a partial response compared with only 4 of 26 (15%) with a score less than or equal to 2. The investigators concluded that there is a possible association between a higher mononuclear inflammatory density score and response but that the numbers of patients to date are too small to make any definitive conclusions. Ongoing larger phase III studies should provide more clarity.

Gene Signatures

KEYNOTE-012 also sought to determine if the use of a 6-gene signature of IFN-γ–related genes that was previously identified to predict response in melanoma studies could be predictive of response to pembrolizumab in patients with GE tumors.[20] The 6 genes (CXCL9, CXCL10, IDO1, IFNG, HLA-DRA, and STAT-1) and an IFN-γ composite score was calculated. Unfortunately, the numbers enrolled were small and the prespecified gene signature did not meet significance at 0.05.

EFFICACY OF PROGRAMMED DEATH-1/PROGRAMMED DEATH LIGAND 1 INHIBITORS IN GASTROESOPHAGEAL CANCER
Pembrolizumab (Programmed Death-1 Inhibitor)

The KEYNOTE-012 study was a multicenter, open-label, phase 1b trial with multiple disease cohorts that enrolled patients with PD-L1$^+$ recurrent/metastatic gastric/GEJ adenocarcinoma.[18] Patients received pembrolizumab, 10 mg/kg, once every 2 weeks for 24 months or until evidence of disease progression. In total, 39 patients were enrolled at 13 centers based in the Untied States, Israel, Japan, South Korea, and Taiwan, and 36 were considered evaluable. A partial response rate of 22% (8/36; 95% CI, 10–39) was observed in this group of heavily pretreated patients, of whom more than 75% had 2 or more prior therapies in the metastatic setting. The regimen was well tolerated, with 13% of patients experiencing grade 3 to 4 toxicity but no patients discontinued the study because of a treatment-related adverse event. PD-L1 positivity has been reported in 40% of gastric tumors and is defined as membranous staining greater than 1% of scorable cells or the presence of a distinctive interface pattern using immunohistochemistry.[15] Although EBV positivity was not assessed in this study, it is plausible that this would influence responsiveness to pembrolizumab due to the role it plays in increasing mutation rates and neoepitope formation.

The KEYNOTE-028 study evaluated the role of pembrolizumab (10 mg/kg every 2 weeks up to 2 years or until progression) in PD-L1$^+$ advanced solid tumors, including esophageal/GEJ cancers (adenocarcinoma and squamous cell cancer [SCC]).[21] At the time of reporting, there were 23 patients enrolled with median follow-up duration of 31 weeks (range: 5.7–71) and 87% had received greater than or equal to 2 prior therapies. Objective response rate was 30% (95% CI, 13.2–52.9) with 6-month and 12-month progression free survival (PFS) rates of 30.4% and 21.7%, respectively.

Efforts to improve responses to PD-1 therapy have included combination therapy with cytotoxic chemotherapy. The KEYNOTE-059 study is a phase II study involving patients with HER2$^-$ advanced gastric/GEJ adenocarcinoma in the first-line setting. Patients received pembrolizumab, 200 mg + fluorouracil (5-FU) 800 mg/m^2 (or capecitabine 1000 mg/m^2 in Japan) + cisplatin 80 mg/m^2, every 3 weeks for 6 cycles followed by pembrolizumab + 5-FU/capecitabine maintenance for up to 2 years or until progression.[22] After median follow-up of 5.5 months (range, 4.0–7.3), 17 patients (94%) had experienced a treatment-related adverse event (any grade), including anorexia, nausea, and neutropenia, of whom 12 patients (67%) experienced grade 3 to 4 toxicities. These preliminary data suggest that combinatorial PD-1/chemotherapy therapy has manageable toxicity profiles in patients with advanced gastric cancer but more mature data are required.

The ongoing phase III study, KEYNOTE-061, compares pembrolizumab versus paclitaxel in patients with advanced gastric cancer in the second line setting.[23]

Patients who progressed on platinum/fluoropyrimidine containing chemotherapy (and HER2 targeting therapy if HER2+) are eligible and are randomized to receive pembrolizumab, 200 mg every 3 weeks, or paclitaxel, 80 mg/m^2, days 1, 8, and 15 of a 28-day cycle. Treatment continues until progression or not tolerated and primary efficacy endpoints are PFS and OS in patients with PD-L1+ tumors.

Nivolumab (Programmed Death-1 Inhibitor)

The CHECKMATE-032 study is a randomized, open-label study, which accrued patients with varying types of advanced solid tumors, including gastric/GEJ tumors to receive nivolumab alone or in combination with ipilimumab (NCT01928394). This study enrolled 160 patients with advanced/metastatic gastric cancer who had progressed on standard chemotherapy, most of whom received greater than or equal to 2 prior regimens.[24] Patients were randomized to receive nivolumab, 3 mg/kg, every 2 weeks (N3); nivolumab, 1 mg/kg, + ipilimumab, 3 mg/kg (N1 + I3); or nivolumab, 3 mg/kg, + ipilimumab, 1 mg/kg (N3 + I1), every 3 weeks for 4 cycles, followed by nivolumab, 3 mg/kg, every 2 weeks, until disease progression or treatment was no longer tolerable. Treatment toxicities (any grade) were more common in the N1 + I3 arm (84%) than the N3 (70%) or N3 + I1 arms (75%). At the time of reporting, 96% (154) patients were evaluable for efficacy outcome reporting and the objective response rates in unselected patients were 14% (nivolumab alone), 26% (N1 + I3), and 10% (N3 + I1). Median OS was highest in the N1 + I3 group (6.9 months; 95% CI, 3.6 — not achieved), followed by N3 (5.0 months; 95% CI, 3.4–12.4) and N3 + I1 (4.8 months; 95% CI, 3.0–9.1). In patients who were PD-L1+, defined as greater than 1% of cells staining positive, response rate for single-agent nivolumab was 27% (4/15) and for the combination of the more active N1/I3 it was an impressive 44% (4/9). For PD-L1− patients, less than 1% response rate for nivolumab was 12% (3/25) and for N1/I3 was 21% (6/29). These data are intriguing and demonstrate that although PD-L1 status should not be used to select for treatment, it may help design future studies where it may be more appropriate for patients who are PD-L1− to be assigned to combination strategies.

Targeting PD-1 with nivolumab has also been shown to have promising efficacy in patients with advanced esophageal SCC. In the ONO-4538 study, nivolumab (3 mg/kg every 2 weeks) was administered to 65 patients in a phase II, single-arm, multicenter study in Japan and found that 17.2% % of patients achieved an objective response.[25] The median OS was 12.1 months and serious adverse events occurred in 14% of patients but no treatment-related deaths occurred. This study supports further phase III testing of nivolumab in patients with advanced esophageal SCC.

Avelumab (Programmed Death Ligand 1 Inhibitor)

Avelumab is a fully human anti–PD-L1 IgG1 antibody currently being studied in multiple tumor types. The JAVELIN study (solid tumor cohort, NCT01772004) was an open-label study with a dose escalation component designed to investigate the safety, tolerability, and clinical activity of avelumab in metastatic/locally advanced solid tumors with expansion cohorts for selected tumor types, including gastric/GEJ tumors.[26] Patients received avelumab, 10 mg/kg, every 2 weeks until progression and treatment-related adverse events occurred in 58.9% patients, of which 9.9% were greater than or equal to grade 3 (fatigue and nausea were most common). Preliminary data show a 9.7% response rate in the second-line setting. In Japanese-only patients who had progressed on prior chemotherapy, the reported overall response rate was 15% (3/20) with the proportion of patients' PFS at 12 weeks 43.3%.[27] The JAVELIN

Gastric 300 trial is currently recruiting patients with recurrent, locally advanced, or metastatic gastric/GEJ tumors in an open-label study comparing avelumab to best supportive care in the third-line setting (NCT02625623). The role of maintenance immunotherapy is being studied in the JAVELIN Gastric 100 study, which compares maintenance treatment comprising single-agent avelumab to continuation of first-line chemotherapy (NCT02625610).[28] During the induction phase, patients receive chemotherapy (5-FU/leucovorin or capecitabine + oxaliplatin) for 12 weeks followed by continuation of chemotherapy or avelumab, 10 mg/kg, every 2 weeks. Primary endpoints are OS and PFS.

Durvalumab (Programmed Death Ligand 1 Inhibitor)

Durvalumab is a selective, high-affinity, human IgG1κ monoclonal antibody that blocks PD-L1 binding to CD80 and PD-1. Single-agent durvalumab, 10 mg/kg intravenously [IV] given every 2 weeks for 12 months, showed potential clinical activity in GE cancers.[29] Trials are currently ongoing investigating the efficacy of durvalumab in advanced GE cancers. A small 26-patient phase II open-label study is currently investigating durvalumab, 1500 mg IV every 4 weeks, for patients with persistent residual esophageal cancer after definitive surgery after concurrent chemoradiation (NCT02639065). A phase Ib/II study is currently enrolling patients in the second-line and third-line metastatic setting with GEJ or gastric adenocarcinomas, to either single-agent durvalumab, single-agent tremelimumab, or the combination durvalumab and tremelimumab (anti–CTLA-4).[30]

EFFICACY OF CYTOTOXIC T-LYMPHOCYTE ASSOCIATED-4 INHIBITORS IN GASTROESOPHAGEAL CANCER
Ipilimumab or Tremelimumab

A randomized phase II trial has investigated the efficacy of sequential ipilimumab versus best supportive care after first-line chemotherapy in patients with metastatic gastric or GEJ cancers.[31] The study did not demonstrate an immune related PFS benefit in favor of ipilimumab (2.92 months vs 4.9 months, hazard ratio [HR] 1.44) with comparable OS (HR 0.87). There have been case reports of response to single-agent tremelimumab, which can be durable, but it is likely this will be in a small minority of patients. It is anticipated that the role of CTLA-4 inhibitors in GE cancer will be as part of combination strategies rather than as single agents. Selected ongoing combination studies are listed in **Tables 1–3**. **Table 4** highlights key ongoing phase III trials and published data from phase I/II studies.

ADJUVANT STUDIES

CheckMate 577 is a randomized phase III study of adjuvant nivolumab in subjects with resected lower esophageal/GE cancer. At the time of writing, accrual has just started and it is anticipated that 760 patients will be randomized in a 2:1 fashion to either nivolumab, 240 mg IV every 2 weeks × 16 weeks, then 480 mg every 4 weeks, for a maximum of 12 months or to the current standard of care (placebo). This is the largest adjuvant study of a checkpoint inhibitor performed to date in esophageal cancer. Primary endpoints are OF and disease-free survival. Results of this study are eagerly anticipated because the lack of data for adjuvant chemotherapy after trimodality therapy in resected stage II/III esophageal cancer has led to confusion about the optimal treatment strategy in patients who fail to achieve a pathologic complete response to neoadjuvant chemoradiation.

Table 1
Selected ongoing clinical trials involving PD-1 targeting therapies for gastroesophageal cancer

Identifier	Phase	Description	Indication	1° Endpoints
Pembrolizumab				
NCT02443324	1	P + ramucirumab	Gastric/GEJ + other tumor types	Safety
NCT02346955	1	P + CM-24 (anti-CEACAM1)	Gastric/GEJ + other tumor types	RP2D, safety
NCT02268825	1	P + FOLFOX chemotherapy	Metastatic gastric/esophageal	Safety
NCT02563548	1b	P + PEGPH20	Gastric/GEJ + other tumor types, second-line	ORR, safety
NCT02689284	1b/2	P + margetuximab (anti-HER2)	Metastatic, HER2$^+$, second-line	MTD, antitumor activity
NCT02730546	1/2	P + chemotherapy + RT	Resectable GEJ/cardia	Pathologic response, PFS
NCT02452424	1/2	P + PLX3397 (CSF1R inhibitor)	Gastric + other tumor types	Safety
NCT02318901	1/2	P + trastuzumab/emtansine/cetuximab	HER2$^+$ gastric + other tumor types	R2PD
NCT02393248	1/2	P or chemotherapy + INCB054828 (anti-FGR)	Multiple lines, gastric/GEJ	Safety, MTD
NCT02335411	2	P ± chemotherapy (KEYNOTE-059)	Multiple lines, gastric/GEJ	Safety, ORR
NCT02830594	2	P + RT	Multiple lines, metastatic gastric/GEJ	Biomarkers
NCT02494583	3	P ± chemotherapy (cisplatin + 5-FU/capecitabine)	Metastatic, first line	PFS, OS
NCT02370498	3	P vs paclitaxel (KEYNOTE-061)	Second-line gastric/GEJ	PFS, OS
Nivolumab (N)				
NCT02746796	2	N + chemotherapy	First-line gastric/GEJ	ORR
NCT02267343	3	N vs placebo	Unresectable gastric/GEJ	OS

Abbreviations: CEACAM1, carcinoembryonic antigen-related cell adhesion molecule 1; CM, anti-CEACAM1 antibody; CSF1R, colony stimulating factor 1 receptor; FGR, fibroblast growth factor; MTD, maximum tolerated dose; N, nivolumab; ORR, objective response rate; P, pembrolizumab; R2PD, recommended phase 2 dose; RT, radiation therapy.

Table 2
Selected ongoing clinical trials involving PD-L1 and CTLA-4 targeting therapies for gastroesophageal cancer

Identifier	Phase	Description	Indication	1° Endpoints
Durvalumab				
NCT02572687	1	D + ramucirumab	Second-line/subsequent-line gastric/GEJ	Safety
NCT02734004	1/2	D + olaparib	Advanced ATM-negative gastric cancer	Disease control rate, safety.
NCT02318277	1/2	D + epacadostat (IDO inhibitor)	Second-line/subsequent-line gastric/GEJ	Safety, ORR
NCT02678182	2	D vs capecitabine vs trastuzumab vs control	Locally advanced/metastatic HER2 ± gastric cancer, maintenance therapy	PFS
Avelumab				
NCT01772004	1	A monotherapy	First-line maintenance, second-line gastric/GEJ	Safety, ORR
NCT02625623	3	A vs best supportive care	Third-line gastric/GEJ cancer	OS
NCT02625610	3	A vs chemotherapy	Continuation 1st line therapy metastatic/unresectable gastric/GEJ	PFS, OS
Ipilimumab				
NCT01585987	2	I vs best supportive care	Maintenance after first-line therapy, gastric/GEJ	immune related PFS

Abbreviations: A, avelumab; ATM, ataxia telangiectasia mutated protein; D, durvalumab; I, ipilimumab; IDO, indoleamine 2; 3-dihydrogenase; ORR, objective response rate.

Table 3
Selected ongoing clinical trials of combinatorial immune checkpoint regimens for gastroesophageal cancer

Identifier	Phase	Description	Indication	1° Endpoints
NCT02834013	2	Nivolumab + ipilimumab	Metastatic gastric SCC, multiple lines, other tumor types	ORR
NCT01928394	1/2	Nivolumab ± ipilimumab	Gastric + other tumor types, multiple lines	ORR
NCT02488759	1/2	Nivolumab ± ipilimumab	EBV + gastric cancer (neoadjuvant + metastatic)	Safety, ORR,
NCT02340975	1b/2	Durvalumab + tremelimumab	Multiple lines, metastatic gastric/GEJ	Safety, ORR, PFS
NCT02658214	1b	Durvalumab + tremelimumab + chemotherapy	Gastric/GEJ + other tumor types, multiple lines	Safety
NCT02735239	1/2	Durvalumab + tremelimumab ± oxaliplatin/ capecitabine ± RT	Multiple lines esophageal/GEJ	Safety

Abbreviations: ORR, objective response rate; RT, radiation therapy.

Table 4
Summary of selected ongoing phase III or completed phase 1/2 trials in refractory setting in gastroesophageal cancer

Anti–PD-1 or Anti–PD-L1 or Anti–CTLA-4	Adjuvant or Neoadjuvant	First-Line Metastatic	Second-Line Metastatic	Refractory Disease (Phase 1/2 Trials)
Nivolumab (PD-1)	CheckMate 577 (PIII) Nivolumab vs placebo in resected stage II/III E/GEJ	In development		CheckMate 032 (PI/II) ORR 14% PD-L1 unselected ORR 27% PD-L1 +ve (>1%) ONO-4538 (PII) ORR 17.2% (Asian patients, squamous cell esophageal)
Pembrolizumab (PD-1)		KEYNOTE-059 (PII) Pembro + cis/5-FU (cohort B) or pembro alone (cohort C) KEYNOTE-062 (PIII) Pembrolizumab vs pembrolizumab + cis/5-FU vs placebo + cis/5-FU	KEYNOTE-061 (PIII) Pembro vs paclitaxel KEYNOTE-181 (PIII) Pembro vs paclitaxel, docetaxel or irinotecan	KEYNOTE-012 (PI) ORR 22% KEYNOTE-028 (PI) ORR 30% KEYNOTE-180 (PII) Third-line study of single-agent pembrolizumab
Avelumab (PD-L1)		JAVELIN Gastric 100 (PIII) Maintenance svelumab after FOLFOX		JAVELIN (PI) ORR 9.7% PD-L1 unselected ORR 18.2% PD-L1 +ve (>1%)
Nivolumab/ipilimumab				CheckMate 032 (PI/II) ORR 26% PD-L1 unselected ORR 44% PD-L1 +ve (>1%)
Durvalumab/tremelimumab				NCT02340975 (PI/II) Durvalumab vs tremelimumab vs combination

Abbreviations: +ve, positive; cis, cisplatin; E,esophageal; EGI, esophagogastric junction; ORR: objective response rate; PII, phase 2; PIII, phase 3.

SUMMARY

The diversity of clinical outcomes seen in patients with similar stages of GE cancer cannot be explained by molecular heterogeneity alone. Although tumor mutational burden and MSI status have been shown to be predictive of response to checkpoint inhibitors in NSCLC and colorectal cancer, respectively, it is likely that additional differences in density of TIL and PD-L1 and EBV expression also play a significant role in upper GI tumors. The role of how immunosuppressive factors like myeloid-derived suppressor cells, $CD4^+CD25^+$ $FoxP3^+$ regulatory T cells and indoleamine 2,3-dioxygenase interact in the immune microenvironment needs to be elucidated. It is likely that GE tumors identified with an adaptive immune resistance pattern with $CD8^+$ T cell–infiltrated tumors containing high presence of PD-L1 expression are more likely to respond to single-agent PD-1 inhibition and may be the 14% to 17% of tumors that have been identified as responding in unselected patients. A greater understanding is needed as to why esophageal adenocarcinomas harbor at least 2 checkpoints, with PD-L1 and PD-L2 reported. It must be asked if tumor location plays a role with perhaps distinctive biology emerging between esophageal, GEJ, and gastric cardia tumors. A thorough evaluation of other checkpoints in addition to a greater understanding of the immune milieu is needed if optimal clinical trials are to be designed. Continuing efforts to identify predictive signatures that can guide treatment decisions and refine PD-L1 assessment so that it becomes easier to interpret are needed. In 2016, it is known that the higher the PD-L1 expression the higher the response rate, and this seems similar for combination strategies involving PD-1/CTLA-4 inhibitors. There are, however, a significant subset of PD-L1$^-$ patients responding to

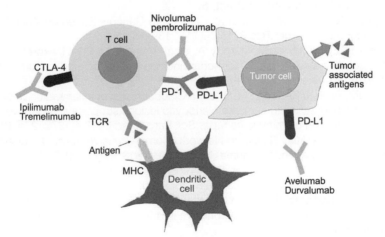

Fig. 1. Components of immune system relevant to GE cancer therapy. T cells express CTLA-4 antigens on their cell surface, which down-regulate T cell functions. Anti-CTLA4 antibodies (ipilimumab and tremilumumab) can bind to CTLA-4 receptors on T cells and reverse their immunosuppressive T cell functions. PD-1 receptors on T cells bind to PD-L1 and PD-L2 ligands on tumor cell surfaces. Anti–PD-1 antibodies (nivolumab and pembrolizumab) bind to PD-1 receptors preventing their interactions with its ligands. Similarly, anti–PD-L1 antibodies (avelumab and durvalumab) bind to PD-L1 receptors, preventing their interaction with PD-1 receptors. Tumors express specific antigens, which can activate antigen presenting cells (dendritic cells) by binding to major histocompatibility complex (MHC) receptors, which bind to T-cell receptors (TCR) on T-cell surfaces. This results in T-cell activation and differentiation, which can ultimately result in B-cell activation and antibody production.

combination strategies, with 21% of heavily pretreated patients responding to nivolumab/ipilimumab combinations.

There may not be a significant difference in PD-L1 expression between stages of disease at presentation, indicating that checkpoint inhibition may have activity in early-stage as well as late-stage disease. The ongoing CheckMate 577 study of adjuvant nivolumab is expected to complete accrual in 2017, with some early results available in 2019. As the data from these larger studies become available, they will provide a more nuanced understanding of the immunologic interactions that are occurring in the microenvironment of GE cancer and it is hoped provide further targets for immune-based therapy (**Fig. 1**).

REFERENCES

1. Van Cutsem E, Moiseyenko VM, Tjulandin S, et al. Phase III study of docetaxel and cisplatin plus fluorouracil compared with cisplatin and fluorouracil as first-line therapy for advanced gastric cancer: a report of the V325 Study Group. J Clin Oncol 2006;24(31):4991–7.

2. Al-Batran SE, Hartmann JT, Probst S, et al. Phase III trial in metastatic gastro-esophageal adenocarcinoma with fluorouracil, leucovorin plus either oxaliplatin or cisplatin: a study of the Arbeitsgemeinschaft Internistische Onkologie. J Clin Oncol 2008;26(9):1435–42.

3. Kang YK, Shah MA, Ohtsu A, et al. A randomized, open-label, multicenter, adaptive phase 2/3 study of trastuzumab emtansine (T-DM1) versus a taxane (TAX) in patients (pts) with previously treated HER2-positive locally advanced or metastatic gastric/gastroesophageal junction adenocarcinoma (LA/MGC/GEJC). J Clin Oncol 2016;34(suppl 4S) [abstract: 5].

4. Teng MW, Ngiow SF, Ribas A, et al. Classifying Cancers Based on T-cell Infiltration and PD-L1. Cancer Res 2015;75(11):2139–45.

5. Thompson ED, Zahurak M, Murphy A, et al. Patterns of PD-L1 expression and CD8 T cell infiltration in gastric adenocarcinomas and associated immune stroma. Gut 2016. [Epub ahead of print].

6. Taube JM, Anders RA, Young GD, et al. Colocalization of inflammatory response with B7-h1 expression in human melanocytic lesions supports an adaptive resistance mechanism of immune escape. Sci Transl Med 2012;4(127):127ra137.

7. Cancer Genome Atlas Research Network. Comprehensive molecular characterization of gastric adenocarcinoma. Nature 2014;513(7517):202–9.

8. Le DT, Uram JN, Wang H, et al. PD-1 blockade in tumors with mismatch-repair deficiency. N Engl J Med 2015;372(26):2509–20.

9. Spranger S, Spaapen RM, Zha Y, et al. Up-regulation of PD-L1, IDO, and T(regs) in the melanoma tumor microenvironment is driven by CD8(+) T cells. Sci Transl Med 2013;5(200):200ra116.

10. Alexandrov LB, Nik-Zainal S, Wedge DC, et al. Signatures of mutational processes in human cancer. Nature 2013;500(7463):415–21.

11. Moons LM, Kusters JG, Bultman E, et al. Barrett's oesophagus is characterized by a predominantly humoral inflammatory response. J Pathol 2005;207(3):269–76.

12. Fitzgerald RC, Abdalla S, Onwuegbusi BA, et al. Inflammatory gradient in Barrett's oesophagus: implications for disease complications. Gut 2002;51(3):316–22.

13. Llosa NJ, Cruise M, Tam A, et al. The vigorous immune microenvironment of microsatellite instable colon cancer is balanced by multiple counter-inhibitory checkpoints. Cancer Discov 2015;5(1):43–51.

14. Giampieri R, Maccaroni E, Mandolesi A, et al. Mismatch repair deficiency may affect clinical outcome through immune response activation in metastatic gastric cancer patients receiving first-line chemotherapy. Gastric Cancer 2016;20(1): 156–63.

15. Wu C, Zhu Y, Jiang J, et al. Immunohistochemical localization of programmed death-1 ligand-1 (PD-L1) in gastric carcinoma and its clinical significance. Acta Histochem 2006;108(1):19–24.

16. Hou J, Yu Z, Xiang R, et al. Correlation between infiltration of FOXP3+ regulatory T cells and expression of B7-H1 in the tumor tissues of gastric cancer. Exp Mol Pathol 2014;96(3):284–91.

17. Geng Y, Wang H, Lu C, et al. Expression of costimulatory molecules B7-H1, B7-H4 and Foxp3+ Tregs in gastric cancer and its clinical significance. Int J Clin Oncol 2015;20(2):273–81.

18. Muro K, Chung HC, Shankaran V, et al. Pembrolizumab for patients with PD-L1-positive advanced gastric cancer (KEYNOTE-012): a multicentre, open-label, phase 1b trial. Lancet Oncol 2016;17(6):717–26.

19. Derks S, Nason KS, Liao X, et al. Epithelial PD-L2 expression marks barrett's esophagus and esophageal adenocarcinoma. Cancer Immunol Res 2015; 3(10):1123–9.

20. Ayers M, Lunceford J, Nebozhyn M, et al. Relationship between immune gene signatures and clinical response to PD-1 blockade with pembrolizumab (MK-3475) in patients with advanced solid tumors. J Immunother Cancer 2015;3(Suppl 2):P80.

21. Doi T, Piha-Paul SA, Jalal SI, et al. Updated results for the advanced esophageal carcinoma cohort of the phase Ib KEYNOTE-028 study of pembrolizumab (MK-3475). J Clin Oncol 2016;34(Suppl 4S) [abstract: 7].

22. Fuchs CS, Ohtsu A, Tabernero J, et al. Preliminary safety data from KEYNOTE-059: Pembrolizumab plus 5-fluorouracil (5-FU) and cisplatin for first-line treatment of advanced gastric cancer. J Clin Oncol 2016;34(15_suppl 4037).

23. Ohtsu A, Tabernero J, Bang YJ, et al. Pembrolizumab (MK-3475) versus paclitaxel as second-line therapy for advanced gastric or gastroesophageal junction (GEJ) adenocarcinoma: Phase 3 KEYNOTE-061 study. J Clin Oncol 2016; 34(suppl 4S) [abstract: TPS183].

24. Janjigian YY, Bendell JC, Calvo E, et al. CheckMate-032: Phase I/II, open-label study of safety and activity of nivolumab (nivo) alone or with ipilimumab (ipi) in advanced and metastatic (A/M) gastric cancer (GC). 2016;34(suppl):[abstract: 4010].

25. Kojima T, Hara H, Yamaguchi K, et al Phase II study of nivolumab (ONO-4538/BMS-936558) in patients with esophageal cancer: preliminary report of overall survival. 2016;34(suppl 4S):[abstract: TPS175].

26. Kelly K, Patel MR, Infante JR, et al. Avelumab (MSB0010718C), an anti-PD-L1 antibody, in patients with metastatic or locally advanced solid tumors: assessment of safety and tolerability in a phase I, open-label expansion study. J Clin Oncol 2015;33(suppl) [abstract: 3044].

27. Nishina T, SK, Iwasa S, et al. Safety, PD-L1 expression, and clinical activity of avelumab (MSB0010718C), an anti-PD-L1 antibody, in Japanese patients with advanced gastric or gastroesophageal junction cancer. J Clin Oncol 2016; 34(suppl 4S) [abstract: 168].

28. Moehler MH, TJ, Gurtler JS, et al. Maintenance therapy with avelumab (MSB0010718C; anti-PD-L1) vs continuation of first-line chemotherapy in patients with unresectable, locally advanced or metastatic gastric cancer: the phase 3 JAVELIN Gastric 100 trial. J Clinoncol 2016;34(suppl) [abstract: TPS4134].

29. Segal NH, ASJ, Brahmer JR, et al. Preliminary data from a multi-arm expansion study of MEDI4736, an anti-PD-L1 antibody. J Clin Oncol 2014;32(suppl):5s [abstract: 3002].

30. Kelly RJ, Chung K, Yu G, et al. Phase Ib/II study to evaluate the safety and anti-tumor activity of durvalumab (MEDI4736) and tremelimumab as monotherapy or in combination, in patients with recurrent or metastatic gastric/gastroesophageal junction adenocarcinoma. J Immunother Cancer 2015;3(Suppl 2):P157.

31. Moehler MH, CJY, Kim YH, et al. A randomized, open-label, two-arm phase II trial comparing the efficacy of sequential ipilimumab (ipi) versus best supportive care (BSC) following first-line (1L) chemotherapy in patients with unresectable, locally advanced/metastatic (A/M) gastric or gastro-esophageal junction (G/GEJ) cancer. J Clin Oncol 2016;4(suppl) [abstract: 4011].

Antiangiogenic Therapy in Gastroesophageal Cancer

Zhaohui Jin, MD, Harry H. Yoon, MD, MHS*

KEYWORDS

- Angiogenesis • Gastric cancer • Esophageal cancer • Immunotherapy
- Checkpoint inhibitor

KEY POINTS

- Antiangiogenesis therapy is one of only 2 biologically targeted approaches (the other being anti–human epidermal growth factor receptor 2 [HER2] therapy) shown to improve overall survival over standard of care in advanced adenocarcinoma of the stomach or gastroesophageal junction (GEJ).
- Therapeutic targeting of vascular endothelial growth factor receptor 2, either its extracellular domain (ramucirumab) or tyrosine kinase domain (apatinib), has been demonstrated to improve overall survival in patients with previously treated advanced gastric/GEJ adenocarcinoma.
- To date, no antiangiogenesis therapy has demonstrated an overall survival benefit in patients with chemo-naïve or resectable esophagogastric cancer or in patients whose tumors arise from the esophagus.
- Promising clinical investigations include the combination of antiangiogenesis therapy with immune checkpoint inhibition and anti-HER2 therapy.

INTRODUCTION

Gastric and esophageal cancers are the fifth and eighth most common malignancies worldwide, respectively, with a combined global incidence of 1.4 million cases yearly.[1] In the United States, an estimated 43,280 new cases and 26,420 deaths from gastroesophageal cancer will occur in 2016.[2] Prognosis remains poor for this patient population with a 5-year-overall survival (OS) rate of 29% and 20% for gastric and esophageal cancer, respectively, underscoring the need for novel therapies.[3]

Angiogenesis is primarily mediated by the interaction between vascular endothelial growth factor (VEGF) and its receptors and is critical for tumor growth, progression,

Disclosure Statement: Dr H.H. Yoon has received research funding from Lilly, Genentech/Roche, and Merck and has received honoraria for serving on advisory boards for Lilly, Genentech/Roche, and Five Prime.
Department of Medical Oncology, Mayo Clinic, 200 First Street Southwest, Rochester, MN 55905, USA
* Corresponding author.
E-mail address: Yoon.harry@mayo.edu

invasion, and metastasis.[4] Angiogenesis inhibitors have demonstrated generally modest clinical benefit over the standard of care across multiple tumor types (**Fig. 1**).

Antiangiogenesis therapy is one of only 2 biologically targeted approaches (the other being anti–human epidermal growth factor receptor 2 [HER2] therapy) shown to improve OS over the standard of care in patients with adenocarcinoma of the stomach or gastroesophageal junction (GEJ). In this review, the authors discuss the most current clinical data regarding the anticancer activity of antiangiogenesis monoclonal antibodies (mAbs) and tyrosine kinase inhibitors (TKIs) in gastroesophageal cancer. The authors briefly review areas of ongoing clinical/translational research and future directions.

ANGIOGENESIS PATHWAY

The VEGF family consists of 5 members: VEGF-A (thereafter called VEGF), VEGF-B, VEGF-C, VEGF-D, and placental growth factor (PlGF) (**Fig. 2**). Members of the VEGF family show different affinities for one of the 3 VEGF tyrosine kinase receptors: VEGF receptor (VEGFR)-1, VEGFR-2, and VEGFR-3. Several coreceptors, such as heparan sulfate proteoglycans and neuropilins, have been implicated in promoting the activation of VEGFRs.[5] VEGFR-1 can bind VEGF, VEGF-B, and placental growth factor. VEGFR-2 is activated primarily by VEGF but also by proteolytically cleaved forms of VEGF-C and VEGF-D. VEGFR-3 is activated only by VEGF-C and VEGF-D. VEGFR-1 is expressed on endothelial cells, monocytes/macrophages, hematopoietic stem cells, and certain non-endothelial cell types.[6] VEGFR-2 is expressed exclusively on endothelial and hematopoietic cells[7]; a notable exception includes non–small cell lung cancer (NSCLC) whereby tumor cell expression of VEGFR-2 has been detected.[8] Ligand binding to the receptor leads to receptor homo-dimerization/hetero-dimerization and autophosphorylation, which triggers an intracellular signaling cascade.[9]

The progression from normal esophagus to Barrett esophagus, dysplasia, and adenocarcinoma is characterized by neovascularization, with microvessel density, vascular immaturity, and VEGF expression increasing along the cancer progression sequence.[10] VEGFR-2 is strongly expressed on new endothelial cells feeding the Barrett mucosa. VEGF-mediated angiogenesis is more robust in intestinal-type gastric tumors than diffuse-type, and tumors positive for *H pylori* infection show greater vascularity than those from patients who underwent *H pylori* eradication.[11] In gastric cancers, VEGF expression in tumors and/or sera/plasma concentrations have been correlated with stage,[12] vessel involvement,[13] metastasis,[12–14] and shorter survival.[14,15] Adverse associations have also been found in human esophageal cancer, suggesting the importance of the VEGF axis in the progression of this disease.[16]

INHIBITION OF THE VASCULAR ENDOTHELIAL GROWTH FACTOR AXIS VIA MONOCLONAL ANTIBODIES

Therapeutic inhibition of the VEGF/VEGFR-2 interaction has demonstrated benefit in patients with advanced gastroesophageal adenocarcinoma whose tumor has progressed on prior therapy (**Fig. 3**).

Anti–Vascular Endothelial Growth Factor Monoclonal Antibody

Single-arm clinical trials in gastric/GEJ adenocarcinoma combining bevacizumab (a recombinant humanized anti-VEGF mAb) with cisplatin/irinotecan,[17] modified docetaxel/cisplatin/fluorouracil,[18] and docetaxel/oxaliplatin[19] showed promising activity.

The first randomized examination of bevacizumab in gastroesophageal cancer avastin in gastric cancer study (AVAGAST) enrolled 774 treatment-naïve patients with inoperable, locally advanced, or metastatic gastric or GEJ cancer from Asia

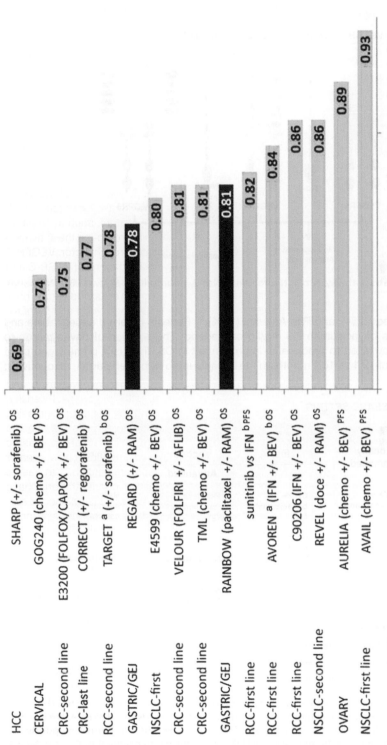

Fig. 1. Incremental gains from antiangiogenesis therapy across multiple tumor types. Hazard ratios for OS are shown from phase 3 trials in Food and Drug Administration–approved indications with a nonbiological agent as a reference arm. Superscripts denote the primary end point. [a] Results censored for subsequent tyrosine kinase inhibitor use[50] or crossover.[51] [b] Crossover permitted. AFLIB, aflibercept; BEV, bevacizumab; CAPOX, capecitabine/oxaliplatin; CRC, colorectal cancer; doce, docetaxel; FOLFIRI, 5-fluorouracil/irinotecan; FOLFOX, fluorouracil plus oxaliplatin; GEJ, gastroesophageal junction; HCC, hepatocellular carcinoma; IFN, interferon; NSCLC, non–small cell lung cancer; PFS, progression-free survival; RAM, ramucirumab; RCC, renal cell carcinoma.

PIGF
VEGF-B
VEGF-A
VEGF-E
VEGF-C
VEGF-D
Extracellular
Cell membrane
Intracellular
Nrp-1
Nrp-2
VEGFR1
VEGFR2
VEGFR3
Vasculogenesis
Angiogenesis
Lymphangiogenesis

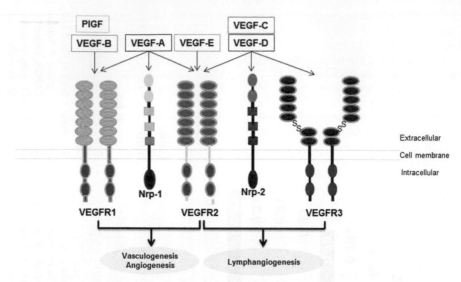

Fig. 2. VEGF axis pathway. Nrp-1, Neuropilin 1; Nrp-2, Neuropilin 2; SS, two disulfide bonds.

(49%), Europe (32%), and Pan-America (19%).[20] Patients received capecitabine and cisplatin plus bevacizumab 7.5 mg/kg or placebo. The addition of bevacizumab to chemotherapy failed to produce an improvement in OS, the trial's primary end point (median OS of 12.1 vs 10.1 months in the bevacizumab vs placebo arms, respectively;

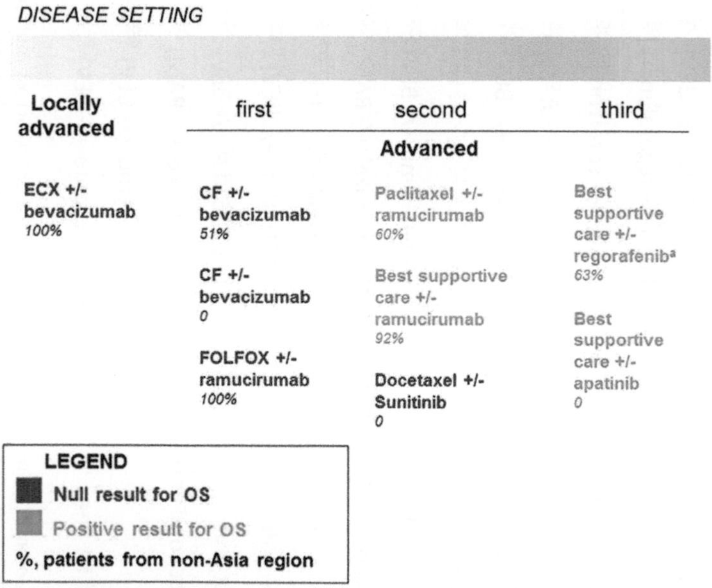

DISEASE SETTING
Locally advanced
first
second
third
Advanced
ECX +/- bevacizumab
100%
CF +/- bevacizumab
51%
CF +/- bevacizumab
0
FOLFOX +/- ramucirumab
100%
Paclitaxel +/- ramucirumab
60%
Best supportive care +/- ramucirumab
92%
Docetaxel +/- Sunitinib
0
Best supportive care +/- regorafenib[a]
63%
Best supportive care +/- apatinib
0
LEGEND
Null result for OS
Positive result for OS
%, patients from non-Asia region

Fig. 3. Benefit from antiangiogenesis therapy over standard of care in gastroesophageal adenocarcinoma has been demonstrated in previously treated advanced disease, not in earlier stages. Results from randomized trials are shown. [a] OS benefit was borderline positive. C, cisplatin; E, epirubicin; F, fluorouracil; FOLFOX, fluorouracil plus oxaliplatin; X, capecitabine.

$P = .1002$). Secondary end points, however, favored the bevacizumab arm, with a median progression-free survival (PFS) of 6.7 months versus 5.3 months ($P = .0037$) and an overall response rate (ORR) of 38.0% versus 29.5% ($P = .0121$), respectively.

An interesting, but not definitively explained, subgroup analysis found that patients from Europe and Pan-America had shorter PFS and OS than Asian patients but derived more benefit from bevacizumab. A lack of bevacizumab benefit in Asian patients was confirmed in a separate study of patients with advanced gastric cancer from Asia (AVATAR).[21] Of note, in AVAGAST, patients from Asia were much more likely to have received second-line therapy ($\sim$60% in Asia vs $\sim$20%–25% in non-Asia), which may have mitigated a potential benefit from bevacizumab. There was no evidence of a differential bevacizumab effect on OS benefit based on histologic subtype (intestinal vs diffuse) or anatomic site of disease (gastric vs GEJ). The results from secondary analysis have spurred interest in examining anti-VEGF axis inhibition within geographic regions.

Anti–Vascular Endothelial Growth Factor Receptor 2 Monoclonal Antibody

Ramucirumab (IMC-1121B) is a fully human recombinant immunoglobulin G1 mAb that specifically and potently inhibits VEGFR-2 by binding to its extracellular domain and inhibits VEGF activities, including receptor phosphorylation and signaling pathway activation.[22]

Second-line setting

Ramucirumab demonstrated improved OS in 2 double-blinded, placebo-controlled, phase 3 trials in previously treated advanced gastric/GEJ adenocarcinoma. In REGARD, 355 patients with metastatic cancer and progression after first-line platinum- and/or fluoropyrimidine-containing regimens were randomized (2:1) to ramucirumab (8 mg/kg every 2 weeks) or placebo. Most patients were from North America, Europe, and Australia. Median OS was statistically significantly higher in ramucirumab-treated patients (5.2 vs 3.8 months, respectively; hazard ratio [HR] 0.776; 95% confidence interval [CI] 0.603–0.998; $P = .0473$).[23] Although overall response rates were similar between arms, ramucirumab-treated patients had improved median PFS (2.1 vs 1.3 months; HR 0.483; $P<.0001$). Ramucirumab was well tolerated.[23] The survival benefit of ramucirumab over best supportive care (BSC) was comparable with that demonstrated by second-line cytotoxic chemotherapy over BSC, making ramucirumab an option for patients who wish to avoid cytotoxic therapy.[24,25]

RAINBOW evaluated the benefit of adding ramucirumab to cytotoxic chemotherapy. In this study, 665 patients with metastatic GEJ/gastric adenocarcinoma were randomized, within 4 months of progression on first-line platinum- and fluoropyrimidine-containing regimens, to paclitaxel combined with ramucirumab (8 mg/kg intravenously [IV] every 2 weeks) or placebo. Ramucirumab-treated patients showed an improvement in the primary end point (median OS 9.6 vs 7.4 months; HR 0.8071; 95% CI 0.678–0.962; $P = .017$). Improvements in PFS and ORR were also statistically significant. Neutropenia was more frequently reported with ramucirumab, but the incidence of febrile neutropenia was comparable between arms.[26]

The results validated the role of therapeutically targeting the VEGFR-2 signaling pathway and led to the first approval of a biological agent in molecularly unselected gastroesophageal cancer.

First-line setting

The effect of adding ramucirumab to front-line chemotherapy was evaluated in a randomized phase 2 US studies of 168 patients with metastatic esophageal, GEJ, or gastric adenocarcinoma. Patients received mFOLFOX6 plus ramucirumab (8 mg/kg IV) or placebo every 14 days. Approximately half the patients had tumors arising from the esophagus, whereas REGARD and RAINBOW did not include these patients. The trial failed to meet its primary end point of PFS (median 6.4 vs 6.7 months in ramucirumab vs placebo, respectively). In an exploratory analysis that attempted to control for a higher premature treatment discontinuation rate in the ramucirumab arm, a longer PFS favoring ramucirumab was observed in the gastric/GEJ cancer subset, whereas no benefit was seen in the esophageal cancer subset.[27] Biomarker analyses are ongoing to further understand these potential tumor site differences. These results have also raised questions regarding the synergy between antiangiogenesis mAbs and fluorouracil plus oxaliplatin (FOLFOX). Consistent with this, negative results were reported in a randomized phase 2 trial (n = 64) evaluating the addition of aflibercept (a recombinant fusion protein that binds VEGF-A, B, and PIGF) to FOLFOX in metastatic esophagogastric adenocarcinoma.[28] A new phase 3 trial (RAINFALL) is examining ramucirumab combined with a different chemotherapy (cisplatin/fluoropyrimidine) in patients with gastric/GEJ adenocarcinoma, excluding tumors arising from the esophagus.

TYROSINE KINASE INHIBITION OF THE VASCULAR ENDOTHELIAL GROWTH FACTOR AXIS

Apatinib in Third-Line Setting

Results from multiple single-arm phase 2 studies examining the VEGFR TKIs sunitinib and sorafenib in advanced gastric/GEJ cancer were mixed.[29–32] However, positive results were reported from a randomized trial examining apatinib. Apatinib is a highly selective and strong inhibitor of VEGFR-2, resulting in a decrease in VEGF-mediated endothelial cell migration, proliferation, and tumor microvascular density. In a phase 3 randomized double-blind trial in patients with chemo-refractory gastric cancer in China, 273 patients who had progressed on second-line therapy were randomly assigned (2:1) to receive apatinib or placebo.[33] Apatinib was associated with an increased median OS (195 days with apatinib vs 140 days with placebo, HR = 0.71, $P<.016$) and improved PFS (78 days vs 53 days, HR = .44, $P<.0001$). The toxicity profile of apatinib was found to be acceptable. Based on these data, apatinib was approved for use by China's Food and Drug Administration (FDA) for metastatic gastric/GEJ adenocarcinoma after second-line chemotherapy. Additional studies to evaluate apatinib in tumors, such as NSCLC and hepatocellular carcinoma, are ongoing.

Regorafenib in Second-/Third-Line Setting

Positive results from a randomized phase 2 trial evaluating regorafenib were recently reported. In this international trial (INTEGRATE; n = 152) patients with advanced gastric/GEJ adenocarcinoma from Australia/New Zealand, South Korea, and Canada were randomized (2:1) to receive BSC plus regorafenib 160 mg or placebo on days 1 to 21 of each 28-day cycle. Patients had tumors refractory to 1 to 2 prior lines of therapy.[34] Median PFS, the primary end point, significantly differed between groups (regorafenib, 2.6 months vs placebo, 0.9 months; HR 0.40; $P<.001$). Interestingly, the effect was greater in South Korea than in other regions (interaction $P<.001$) but consistent across plasma VEGF-A levels. Median OS slightly favored the regorafenib arm (5.8 vs 4.5 months; HR 0.71 [all randomly assigned patients]; stratified log-rank $P = .06$). A phase 3 trial in refractory gastric cancer (INTEGRATE II) is commencing in 2016, and studies evaluating regorafenib with chemotherapy in earlier settings are underway.

LOCALLY ADVANCED DISEASE

Given the activity of antiangiogenesis therapy in advanced disease, an open-label phase 3 trial examined the addition of bevacizumab to perioperative chemotherapy. Patients in the United Kingdom with resectable adenocarcinoma of the stomach, GEJ, or lower esophagus (n = 1062) were randomized (1:1) to standard treatment (3 preoperative and 3 postoperative cycles of epirubicin; cisplatin, capecitabine (ECX) [epirubicin 50 mg/m^2 IV Day 1 (D1), cisplatin 60 mg/m^2 IV D1, and capecitabine 1250 mg/m^2 D1–21] and surgery) or investigational treatment (ECX + bevacizumab 7.5 mg/kg D1 for the 6 cycles followed by 6 maintenance cycles of bevacizumab). Toxicity during chemotherapy was generally similar in both groups.

The trial failed to meet its primary end point of OS (HR 1.06; P = .478; 3-year rates 48.9% in control vs 47.6% in experimental). DFS, pathologic response rates, and curative resection rates (59% control vs 55% experimental) were also similar between groups.[35] The null results, compared with the positive results in second-line advanced disease for ramucirumab, are reminiscent of the discrepant results in resected versus advanced colon cancer, suggesting biological differences impacting the efficacy of antiangiogenesis therapy may exist between gastrointestinal tumors of earlier versus later stage.

ONGOING AREAS OF RESEARCH AND FUTURE DIRECTIONS
Combination with Immune Checkpoint Therapy

Recent studies have revealed a complex relationship between VEGF signaling and anticancer immunity suggesting potential synergy between angiogenesis and immune checkpoint inhibition.

In addition to its critic role in angiogenesis, recent data indicate that VEGF modulates antitumor immunity on multiple levels:

- VEGF induces T regulatory cell proliferation and differentiation, which inhibits effective antitumor response.[36]
- VEGF promotes expansion of myeloid-derived suppressor cells, which are a heterogeneous cell population derived from myeloid cells that inhibit antitumor T-cell response.[37]
- VEGF inhibits antigen-presenting cell (dendritic cell) maturation.[37]
- VEGF inhibits effector T-cell development.[38]
- VEGF suppresses expression of endothelial intercellular adhesion molecule 1 resulting in a dysfunctional tumor vasculature and inhibits tumor infiltration of T cells and other immune effectors.[30]
- VEGF can induce endothelial Fas Ligand (FasL) expression, which leads to apoptosis of tumor-reactive CD8+ T effector cells.[40]

Synergy between VEGF inhibition and immunotherapy was detected in an adoptive T-cell transfer (ACT) mouse model of established B16 melanoma. Administration of VEGF-targeted (but not VEGFR-2-targeted) antibody synergized with ACT to enhance inhibition of tumor growth and prolong survival. Further evaluation showed that anti-VEGF treatment enhanced T-cell infiltration into the tumor.[41] Although PD-1- and VEGFR-2-targeted antibodies, alone or combined, did not affect tumor cell survival in vitro, simultaneous treatment with antiangiogenesis and PD-1 blockade showed synergistic antitumor activity in vivo in a murine colon-26 adenocarcinoma model. Antiangiogenesis therapy did not seem to interfere with PD-1 blockade's enhancement of T-cell infiltration into tumor tissue.[42]

In the clinical setting, combination therapy with antiangiogenesis and immune checkpoint blockade has shown promising results. Compared with ipilimumab monotherapy, combined treatment with ipilimumab and bevacizumab in patients with advanced melanoma induced higher E-selectin expression, morphologic tumor vasculature change, more intense infiltration of CD8+ T cells and CD163+ dendritic macrophages within the tumor vasculature, and increased circulating memory CD4+ and CD8+ cells. The combination therapy led to a median survival of 25.1 months, roughly twice expectation for ipilimumab alone in metastatic melanoma.[43] Combination treatment with atezolizumab (anti-PDL1) and bevacizumab for advanced renal cell cancer showed good safety, promising preliminary clinical effects, and immune modulation of the tumor microenvironment.[44] Multiple trials combining VEGF/VEGFR inhibitors with checkpoint blockade are planned or ongoing (**Table 1**).

Combination with Anti–Human Epidermal Growth Factor Receptor 2 Therapy

Trastuzumab, a humanized mAb, targets the extracellular binding domain of the HER2 receptor and has been approved by the US FDA for the treatment of HER2-positive breast cancer and advanced gastric/GEJ adenocarcinoma. A single-arm phase 2 trial (N = 35) reported promising results from combined trastuzumab, bevacizumab, plus capecitabine/oxaliplatin (CAPOX) in patients with HER2-positive metastatic esophagogastric cancer who had 0 to 1 lines of prior chemotherapy.[45] Therapy was well tolerated. The relative risk was 76.5% by blinded review. Median PFS was 13.9 months and median OS was 26.9 months. These results suggest a possible synergy between anti-VEGF and anti-HER2 therapy in this disease. Trials are underway evaluating the combination of bevacizumab (NCT01359397) or ramucirumab (NCT02726399) with trastuzumab and chemotherapy in HER2-positive advanced gastric cancer.

Predictive Biomarkers

Although no biomarkers that predict benefit from antiangiogenesis therapy have been clinically validated, data from AVAGAST suggested that plasma VEGF-A (measured by enzyme-linked immunosorbent assay) can predict bevacizumab benefit among non-Asian patients with gastric cancer. Patients with higher baseline VEGF-A seemed to benefit from the addition of bevacizumab to chemotherapy (HR 0.72 [95% CI 0.57–0.93]), whereas those with low levels did not (HR 1.01).[46] The value of plasma VEGF-A as a predictive marker was driven by the non-Asia population, in which the HR for OS was 0.59 (interaction $P = .04$) and HR for PFS was 0.54 (interaction $P = .06$). Although interesting, these data need confirmation in future trials.

Attention has also been drawn to *VEGF* gene amplification, which has a frequency of 7% to 12% in human gastric cancers,[47,48] as a possible biomarker. Preclinical and clinical data in HCC suggest that VEGF-A amplification may predict for increased sensitivity to sorafenib.[49] Analysis of tumor samples from a randomized trial of metastatic breast cancer treated with paclitaxel ± bevacizumab suggested that VEGF-A amplification was associated with decreased benefit from bevacizumab. Although major questions remain to be addressed, these data provide a rationale for further study of VEGF-A amplification in esophagogastric cancers.

Most research into predictive antiangiogenesis biomarkers has focused on bevacizumab and multi-target TKIs. Ramucirumab has a different molecular target from bevacizumab, as VEGFR-2 is bound by ligands other than VEGF; it is possible that biomarker analyses in ramucirumab-treated patients may not yield the same results.

Table 1
Ongoing clinical trials studying angiogenesis inhibition in gastroesophageal cancer

Clinical Trial Identifier	Study Medication	Cancer Type	Phase[a]	Sample Size	Comments
Phase 3 trials					
NCT02661971	FLOT with/without ramucirumab	Resectable GC/GEJ	2/3	908	Randomized
NCT02314117	Capecitabine plus cisplatin with/without ramucirumab	Metastatic GC/GEJ	3	616	Randomized, double blinded
NCT02537171	Apatinib 750 mg or 500 mg daily	Advanced GC	3	40	Randomized to 2 different doses
NCT02409199	Apatinib vs docetaxel	Advanced GC	2/3	66	Randomized
NCT02509806	Apatinib as maintenance vs no therapy after first-line chemotherapy	Advanced GC	2/3	48	Randomized
Trials combining angiogenesis inhibition with HER2 or immune checkpoint blockade					
NCT02773524	Regorafenib vs placebo	Refractory advanced GC/EAC	3	350	Randomized
NCT02726399	Ramucirumab plus trastuzumab with capecitabine/cisplatin	Metastatic HER2-positive GC/GEJ	2	37	Nonrandomized
NCT01359397	Bevacizumab plus trastuzumab with docetaxel, oxaliplatin, capecitabine	HER2-positive advanced GC/GEJ	2	—	Nonrandomized
NCT02443324	Ramucirumab plus pembrolizumab	Advanced GC/GEJ, NSCLC, urothelium carcinoma, or biliary tract cancer	1	155	Nonrandomized
NCT02572687	Ramucirumab plus durvalumab	Advanced GC/GEJ, NSCLC, HCC	1	114	Nonrandomized
NCT01633970	Bevacizumab plus atezolizumab with/without chemotherapy	Advanced solid tumor	1	225	Randomized with 6 arms (2 arms include bevacizumab plus atezolizumab with/without FOLFOX)

Abbreviations: EAC, esophageal adenocarcinoma; FLOT, fluorouracil, leucovorin, oxaliplatin, docetaxel; FOLFOX, fluorouracil plus oxaliplatin; GC, gastric cancer; GEJ, gastroesophageal junction cancer; HCC, hepatocellular carcinoma.
[a] Phase designations are based on information provided on clinicaltrials.gov.
Data from ClinicalTrials.gov. US National Institutes of Health (NIH). Available at: https://clinicaltrials.gov/. Accessed July 28, 2016.

REFERENCES

1. Torre LA, Bray F, Siegel RL, et al. Global cancer statistics, 2012. CA Cancer J Clin 2015;65(2):87–108.
2. Siegel RL, Miller KD, Jemal A. Cancer statistics, 2016. CA Cancer J Clin 2016; 66(1):7–30.
3. Siegel RL, Miller KD, Jemal A. Cancer statistics, 2015. CA Cancer J Clin 2015; 65(1):5–29.
4. Kaspar S, Schuler M. Targeted therapies in gastroesophageal cancer. Eur J Cancer 2014;50:1247–58.
5. Kowanetz M, Ferrara N. Vascular endothelial growth factor signaling pathways: therapeutic perspective. Clin Cancer Res 2006;12(17):5018–22.
6. Cross MJ, Dixelius J, Matsumoto T, et al. VEGF-receptor signal transduction. Trends Biochem Sci 2003;28(9):488–94.
7. Millauer B, Wizigmann-Voos S, Schnurch H, et al. High affinity VEGF binding and developmental expression suggest Flk-1 as a major regulator of vasculogenesis and angiogenesis. Cell 1993;72(6):835–46.
8. Holzer TR, Fulford AD, Nedderman DM, et al. Tumor cell expression of vascular endothelial growth factor receptor 2 is an adverse prognostic factor in patients with squamous cell carcinoma of the lung. PLoS One 2013;8(11):e80292.
9. Olsson AK, Dimberg A, Kreuger J, et al. VEGF receptor signalling - in control of vascular function. Nat Rev Mol Cell Biol 2006;7(5):359–71.
10. Lord RV, Park JM, Wickramasinghe K, et al. Vascular endothelial growth factor and basic fibroblast growth factor expression in esophageal adenocarcinoma and Barrett esophagus. J Thorac Cardiovasc Surg 2003;125(2):246–53.
11. Kitadai Y. Cancer-stromal cell interaction and tumor angiogenesis in gastric cancer. Cancer Microenviron 2010;3(1):109–16.
12. Karayiannakis AJ, Syrigos KN, Polychronidis A, et al. Circulating VEGF levels in the serum of gastric cancer patients: correlation with pathological variables, patient survival, and tumor surgery. Ann Surg 2002;236(1):37–42.
13. Maeda K, Chung YS, Ogawa Y, et al. Prognostic value of vascular endothelial growth factor expression in gastric carcinoma. Cancer 1996;77(5):858–63.
14. Yoshikawa T, Tsuburaya A, Kobayashi O, et al. Plasma concentrations of VEGF and bFGF in patients with gastric carcinoma. Cancer Lett 2000;153(1–2):7–12.
15. Chen J, Zhou B, Zhang Y, et al. Clinicopathological and prognostic significance of galectin-1 and vascular endothelial growth factor expression in gastric cancer. World J Gastroenterol 2013;19:2073–9.
16. Shimada H, Takeda A, Nabeya Y, et al. Clinical significance of serum vascular endothelial growth factor in esophageal squamous cell carcinoma. Cancer 2001;92(3):663–9.
17. Shah MA, Ramanathan RK, Ilson DH, et al. Multicenter phase II study of irinotecan, cisplatin, and bevacizumab in patients with metastatic gastric or gastroesophageal junction adenocarcinoma. J Clin Oncol 2006;24(33):5201–6.
18. Shah MA, Jhawer M, Ilson DH, et al. Phase II study of modified docetaxel, cisplatin, and fluorouracil with bevacizumab in patients with metastatic gastroesophageal adenocarcinoma. J Clin Oncol 2011;29(7):868–74.
19. El-Rayes BF, Zalupski M, Bekai-Saab T, et al. A phase II study of bevacizumab, oxaliplatin, and docetaxel in locally advanced and metastatic gastric and gastroesophageal junction cancers. Ann Oncol 2010;21(10):1999–2004.
20. Matsuoka T, Yashiro M. Recent advances in the HER2 targeted therapy of gastric cancer. World J Clin Cases 2015;3(1):42–51.

21. Shen L, Li J, Xu J, et al. Bevacizumab plus capecitabine and cisplatin in Chinese patients with inoperable locally advanced or metastatic gastric or gastroesophageal junction cancer: randomized, double-blind, phase III study (AVATAR study). Gastric cancer 2015;18(1):168–76.

22. Spratlin J. Ramucirumab (IMC-1121B): monoclonal antibody inhibition of vascular endothelial growth factor receptor-2. Curr Oncol Rep 2011;13(2):97–102.

23. Fuchs CS, Tomasek J, Yong CJ, et al. Ramucirumab monotherapy for previously treated advanced gastric or gastro-oesophageal junction adenocarcinoma (REGARD): an international, randomised, multicentre, placebo-controlled, phase 3 trial. Lancet 2014;383(9911):31–9.

24. Kang JH, Lee SI, Lim do H, et al. Salvage chemotherapy for pretreated gastric cancer: a randomized phase III trial comparing chemotherapy plus best supportive care with best supportive care alone. J Clin Oncol 2012;30(13):1513–8.

25. Ford HE, Marshall A, Bridgewater JA, et al. Docetaxel versus active symptom control for refractory oesophagogastric adenocarcinoma (COUGAR-02): an open-label, phase 3 randomised controlled trial. Lancet Oncol 2014;15(1):78–86.

26. Wilke H, Muro K, Van Cutsem E, et al. Ramucirumab plus paclitaxel versus placebo plus paclitaxel in patients with previously treated advanced gastric or gastro-oesophageal junction adenocarcinoma (RAINBOW): a double-blind, randomised phase 3 trial. Lancet Oncol 2014;15(11):1224–35.

27. Yoon HH, Bendell JC, Braiteh FS, et al. Ramucirumab (RAM) plus FOLFOX as front-line therapy (Rx) for advanced gastric or esophageal adenocarcinoma (GE-AC): randomized, double-blind, multicenter phase 2 trial. J Clin Oncol 2014;32(Suppl):5s [abstract: 4004].

28. Enzinger PC, McCleary NJ, Zheng H, et al. Multicenter double-blind randomized phase II: FOLFOX + ziv-aflibercept/placebo for patients (pts) with chemo-naive metastatic esophagogastric adenocarcinoma (MEGA). Paper presented at: Gastrointestinal Cancers Symposium 2016; San Francisco, CA, January 21–23, 2016.

29. Bang YJ, Kang YK, Kang WK, et al. Phase II study of sunitinib as second-line treatment for advanced gastric cancer. Invest New Drugs 2011;29(6):1449–58.

30. Yi JH, Lee J, Lee J, et al. Randomised phase II trial of docetaxel and sunitinib in patients with metastatic gastric cancer who were previously treated with fluoropyrimidine and platinum. Br J Cancer 2012;106(9):1469–74.

31. Sun W, Powell M, O'Dwyer PJ, et al. Phase II study of sorafenib in combination with docetaxel and cisplatin in the treatment of metastatic or advanced gastric and gastroesophageal junction adenocarcinoma: ECOG 5203. J Clin Oncol 2010;28(18):2947–51.

32. Martin-Richard M, Gallego R, Pericay C. Multicenter phase II study of oxaliplatin and sorafenib in advanced gastric adenocarcinoma after failure of cisplatin and fluoropyrimidine treatment: a GEMCAD study. Invest New Drugs 2013;31:1573–9.

33. Qin S. Phase III study of apatinib in advanced gastric cancer: a randomized, double-blind, placebo-controlled trial. J Clin Oncol 2014;32(5s) [abstract: 4003].

34. Pavlakis N, Sjoquist KM, Martin AJ, et al. Regorafenib for the treatment of advanced gastric cancer (INTEGRATE): a multinational placebo-controlled phase II trial. J Clin Oncol 2016;34(23):2728–35.

35. Cunningham D, Smyth E, Stenning S, et al. Peri-operative chemotherapy ± bevacizumab for resectable gastro-oesophageal adenocarcinoma: results from the UK Medical Research Council randomised ST03 trial (ISRCTN 46020948). Eur J Cancer 2015;51(Suppl 3):S400 [abstract: 2201].

36. Terme M, Pernot S, Marcheteau E, et al. VEGFA-VEGFR pathway blockade inhibits tumor-induced regulatory T-cell proliferation in colorectal cancer. Cancer Res 2013;73(2):539–49.
37. Gabrilovich D, Ishida T, Oyama T, et al. Vascular endothelial growth factor inhibits the development of dendritic cells and dramatically affects the differentiation of multiple hematopoietic lineages in vivo. Blood 1998;92(11):4150–66.
38. Ohm JE, Gabrilovich DI, Sempowski GD, et al. VEGF inhibits T-cell development and may contribute to tumor-induced immune suppression. Blood 2003;101(12): 4878–86.
39. Griffioen AW, Damen CA, Martinotti S, et al. Endothelial intercellular adhesion molecule-1 expression is suppressed in human malignancies: the role of angiogenic factors. Cancer Res 1996;56(5):1111–7.
40. Motz GT, Santoro SP, Wang LP, et al. Tumor endothelium FasL establishes a selective immune barrier promoting tolerance in tumors. Nat Med 2014;20(6): 607–15.
41. Shrimali RK, Yu Z, Theoret MR, et al. Antiangiogenic agents can increase lymphocyte infiltration into tumor and enhance the effectiveness of adoptive immunotherapy of cancer. Cancer Res 2010;70(15):6171–80.
42. Yasuda S, Sho M, Yamato I, et al. Simultaneous blockade of programmed death 1 and vascular endothelial growth factor receptor 2 (VEGFR2) induces synergistic anti-tumour effect in vivo. Clin Exp Immunol 2013;172(3):500–6.
43. Hodi FS, Lawrence D, Lezcano C, et al. Bevacizumab plus ipilimumab in patients with metastatic melanoma. Cancer Immunol Res 2014;2(7):632–42.
44. Sznol M, McDermott DF, Jones SF, et al. Phase Ib evaluation of MPDL3280A (anti-PDL1) in combination with bevacizumab (bev) in patients (pts) with metastatic renal cell carcinoma (mRCC). Paper presented at: 2015 ASCO Genitourinary Cancer Symposium. Orlando, FL, January 15–17, 2015.
45. Enzinger PC, Abrams TA, Chan JA, et al. Multicenter phase 2: capecitabine (CAP) + oxaliplatin (OX) + bevacizumab (BEV) + trastuzumab (TRAS) for patients (pts) with metastatic esophagogastric cancer (MEGCA). Paper presented at: ASCO Annual Meeting. Chicago, IL, May 29–June 2, 2015.
46. Shah M, Kang Y, Ohtsu A. Tumor and blood plasma biomarker analyses in the AVAGAST phase III randomized study of first-line bevacizumab plus capecitabine/cisplatin in patients with advanced gastric cancer. Ann Oncol 2010;20(8): viii63–77 [abstract: 174PD].
47. Comprehensive molecular characterization of gastric adenocarcinoma. Nature 2014;513(7517):202–9.
48. Andreozzi M, Quagliata L, Gsponer JR, et al. VEGFA gene locus analysis across 80 human tumour types reveals gene amplification in several neoplastic entities. Angiogenesis 2014;17(3):519–27.
49. Horwitz E, Stein I, Andreozzi M, et al. Human and mouse VEGFA-amplified hepatocellular carcinomas are highly sensitive to sorafenib treatment. Cancer Discov 2014;4(6):730–43.
50. Bracarda S, Bellmunt J, Melichar B, et al. Overall survival in patients with metastatic renal cell carcinoma initially treated with bevacizumab plus interferon-alpha2a and subsequent therapy with tyrosine kinase inhibitors: a retrospective analysis of the phase III AVOREN trial. BJU Int 2011;107(2):214–9.
51. Escudier B, Eisen T, Stadler WM, et al. Sorafenib for treatment of renal cell carcinoma: final efficacy and safety results of the phase III treatment approaches in renal cancer global evaluation trial. J Clin Oncol 2009;27(20):3312–8.

Update on Gastroesophageal Adenocarcinoma Targeted Therapies

Steven B. Maron, MD[a], Daniel V.T. Catenacci, MD[b],*

KEYWORDS

- Gastroesophageal • Gastric • MET • Epidermal growth factor receptor • HER2
- ERBB2 • Treatment • Targeted

KEY POINTS

- Trastuzumab is a treatment standard for HER2 amplified/overexpressed gastroesophageal adenocarcinoma, yet benefit has not been demonstrated in second and later lines of therapy, or beyond progression in first line therapy.
- Anti-epidermal growth factor receptor therapy warrants further investigation for gene amplification/over-expression despite lack of benefit demonstrated in unselected gastroesophageal patients to date.
- Anti-MET therapy has not demonstrated benefit in 'over-expressing' gastroesophageal patients in any line of therapy, but evidence supports further investigation in patients with gene amplification/overexpression.

BACKGROUND

Distal gastric adenocarcinoma (GC) incidence remains the fifth most common cancer globally, and the third highest for cancer-related mortality.[1–3] Approximately twenty-five thousand new GC cases and eleven thousand deaths were predicted in the United States in 2015.[4] Further, esophagogastric junction adenocarcinoma (EGJ) incidence is increasing. When assessing GC and EGJ cancers, together known as gastroesophageal cancer (GEC), the majority of patients present with metastatic or locally advanced disease with a high risk of recurrence despite aggressive perioperative therapy. In the metastatic/recurrent setting, median overall survival remains approximately 11 months

Disclosure Statement: D.V.T. Catenacci has received research funding from Genentech/Roche, Amgen, OncoplexDx/Nantomics and honoraria from Genentech/Roche, Amgen, Eli Lilly, Five Prime, OncoplexDx/Nantomics, Guardant Health, Foundation Medicine.
[a] Section of Hematology/Oncology, University of Chicago Comprehensive Cancer Center, 5841 South Maryland Avenue, Chicago, IL 60637, USA; [b] The University of Chicago Medical Center & Biological Sciences, 900 East 57th Street, KCBD Building, Office 7128, Chicago, IL 60637, USA
* Corresponding author.
E-mail address: dcatenac@medicine.bsd.uchicago.edu

Hematol Oncol Clin N Am 31 (2017) 511–527
http://dx.doi.org/10.1016/j.hoc.2017.01.009
0889-8588/17/© 2017 Elsevier Inc. All rights reserved.

hemonc.theclinics.com

with optimal palliative chemotherapy in Erb-B2 receptor tyrosine kinase 2 (ERBB2) non-amplified patients. Over the past decade, molecular subtyping of GEC has highlighted the inter-patient heterogeneity of GEC and uncovered potentially actionable molecular pathways.[5] Routine next generation sequencing identified that at least 37% of GC patients harbor genetic alterations, namely amplifications, in receptor tyrosine kinases (RTKs), including *ERBB2, MET,* epidermal growth factor receptor (*EGFR*), kirsten rat sarcoma 2 viral oncogene homolog (KRAS), and fibroblast growth factor receptor 2 (FGFR2).[6–8] Clinical trials of agents targeting these pathways have had mixed results. However, interpretation of these results requires understanding both the agents used as well as the study population. These genomic events, as well as recently derived key subsets of the disease, namely microsatellite instability-high (MSI-high), EBV-associated (EBV), chromosomal instability (CIN), and genomically stable (GS), provide for more molecularly targeted therapeutic possibilities.[9]

ERBB2

ERBB2, or HER2, is a transmembrane RTK within the EGFR family, encoded at chromosome 17q21. HER2 regulates proliferation, adhesion, differentiation, and migration via activation of the RAS-MAPK and PI3K-AKT pathways (**Fig. 1**). HER2 lacks an exogenous ligand and is transactivated via heterodimerization with other HER family members leading to downstream kinase activation. Significant and therapeutically relevant protein overexpression results predominantly from gene amplification; less commonly, other genomic events may include activating mutation. HER2 immunohistochemistry (IHC) expression localizes to the cell membrane in well-differentiated adenocarcinoma and to the cytoplasm in poorly differentiated adenocarcinomas, which may affect treatment response.[10] *HER2*-amplified tumors are more common

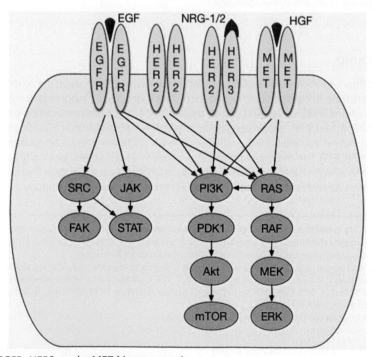

Fig. 1. EGFR, HER2, and c-MET kinase cascade.

with EGJ (15%–32%) compared with the distal GC (10%–15%), and the prognostic impact of *HER2* amplification remains controversial (**Table 1**).[11–15]

Effective targeting of HER2 in GEC was initially demonstrated using trastuzumab, a humanized monoclonal anti-HER2 antibody against the HER2 ectodomain (**Table 2**). The phase III Trastuzumab for Gastric Cancer (ToGA) trial evaluated a first-line fluoro-pyrimidine/cisplatin chemotherapy doublet with or without trastuzumab in patients with HER-2 overexpressing (any IHC 3 + or fluorescence in situ hybridization [FISH] HER2:CEP17 ratio $\geq$2) unresectable or metastatic GEC.[15] Patients receiving trastuzumab survived a median of 13.8 months versus 11.1 months with chemotherapy alone (hazard ratio [HR] 0.74, P = .0046), and response rates were 47% and 35%, respectively, in the intention-to-treat (ITT) population. In a subset analysis, median survival was 16 versus 11.8 months in the combined IHC2 positive/FISH positive and IHC3 positive groups, accounting for 77% of the patients enrolled, whereas IHC0-1 positive/FISH positive patients appeared to derive no benefit. This trial therefore led to the approval of trastuzumab in HER2 overexpressing gastric cancer for the IHC2 positive/FISH positive and IHC3 positive subsets of the trial.[15,16]

Finally, whereas trastuzumab binds domain IV of HER2, pertuzumab binds domain II, and thereby prevents dimerization with other RTKs, namely HER3. The Clinical Evaluation of Pertuzumab and Trastuzumab (CLEOPATRA) trial in breast cancer revealed progression-free and overall survival benefits with the addition of pertuzumab to trastuzumab and chemotherapy as first-line therapy,[17] and initial results from the counterpart (JACOB) A Study of Pertuzumab in Combination With Trastuzumab and Chemotherapy in Participants With Human Epidermal Growth Factor Receptor 2 (HER2)-Positive Metastatic Gastroesophageal Junction or Gastric Cancer.[18] A large trial with appropriate HER2 selection (ie, not allowing IHC0-1+/FISH+ patients) and without the concern of later line evolution (ie, not second or later line of therapy) or lack of antibody-dependent cell-mediated cytotoxicity (ADCC) (ie, like the lapatinib trials) will likely allow JACOB to adequately test the hypothesis whether there is benefit of adding pertuzumab to standard cytotoxic plus trastuzumab therapy for these patients. However, intratumoral and spatial HER2 heterogeneity (at higher rates than compared with breast cancer) may still have implications on the overall trial results. The results of this trial remain eagerly awaited.

Lapatinib, a selective intracellular tyrosine kinase inhibitor (TKI) of ERBB1 and ERBB2 was also studied in first- and second-line GEC (see **Table 2**). The phase III Lapatinib Optimization Study in ErbB2 Positive Gastric Adenocarcinoma (TRIO-013/LOGIC) trial randomized 545 untreated first-line HER2 positive (HER2: CEP17 ratio $\geq$2 by FISH or IHC 3 + if FISH not available) GEC patients to receive capecitabine and oxaliplatin in addition to either lapatinib or placebo. Lapatinib increased objective response from 39% to 53%, and modestly increased median PFS from 5.4 to 6 months, but failed to confer an overall survival benefit in the ITT population.[19] Younger and Asian patients appeared to derive the most benefit in subset analyses. The absolute level of amplification positively correlated with outcome, as previously described,[20,21] signifying heterogeneity of benefit within the current HER2 positive classification. *HER2* amplification varies depending on the report, ranging from 4% to 20% of GEC patients (see **Table 1**). Recently, the degree of amplification has been shown to correlate closely with both absolute protein expression level and clinical benefit.[22] The inter-trial variations in absolute amplification/expression and lapatinib's lack of ADCC as compared with trastuzumab, serve as two of many potential explanations when contrasting outcomes of ToGA and LOGiC.

In the second line, the phase III Asian Tykerb with Taxol in Asian HER2-Positive Gastric Cancer (TyTAN) trial enrolled patients regardless of HER2 expression (FISH ratio $\geq$2 were eligible), where 31% of patients enrolled were IHC 0 to 1 positive/FISH

Table 1
Rates of key receptor tyrosine kinase overexpression and gene amplification in gastroesophageal cancer

Study	ERBB2		EGFR		MET		Population	Site
	Amp (%)	Exp (%)	Amp (%)	Exp (%)	Amp (%)	Exp (%)		
Nagatsuma et al,[43] 2015	9	11.8	2.4	24.9	1.3	24.9	950	Gastric, resected
Nakajima et al,[64] 1999	11.7	16.4	—	—	10.2	46.1	128	Gastric, resected
Lennerz et al,[44] 2011	8.9	—	4.7	—	2	—	489	Gastroesophageal, all comers
Terashima et al,[13] 2012	13.3	13.6	—	9	—	—	829	Gastric, resected
Van Cutsem et al,[85] 2015	4.1	21.4/32.2 (G/EGJ)	—	—	—	—	3280	Gastric/EGJ, advanced
Kim et al,[41] 2008	—	—	2.3	27.4	—	—	511	Gastric, resected
Luber et al,[57] 2011	—	—	3	—	—	—	39	Gastric/EGJ, advanced
Petty et al,[58] 2014	—	—	6.1	—	—	—	450	Esophageal/EGJ, advanced
Catenacci et al,[61] 2015	—	—	—	—	5.2	35.2	394	Gastroesophageal, resected
Graziano et al,[66] 2011	—	—	—	—	10	—	216	Gastric, resected
Lee et al,[65] 2012	—	—	—	—	3.4	62.3	439	Gastric, resected
Jardim et al,[73] 2014	—	—	—	—	6	—	77	Gastroesophageal, all comers

Abbreviations: Amp, amplification; Exp, overexpression.

Table 2
HER2-directed phase III clinical trials for gastroesophageal cancer

Line	Trial	N	Treatment	Primary Endpoint (Met?)	mOS (mo)	HR	mPFS (mo)	HR	RR (%)
1L	Bang et al,[15] 2010 TOGA	584	Cis/FP	OS (Yes)	11.8[a]	0.74	5.5	0.71	35
			Cis/FP + Trastuzumab		16[a]	0.65[a] P<.05[a]	6.7	P<.001	47
1L	Hecht et al,[19] 2016 LOGiC	545 (487)	Cis/FP	OS (No)	10.5	0.91	5.4	0.82	39
			Cis/FP + Lapatinib		12.2	P = N.S.	6	P = .03	53
2L	Satoh et al,[23] 2014 TYTAN	261	Paclitaxel	OS (No)	8.9	0.84	4.4	0.84	9
			Paclitaxel + Lapatinib		11	P = N.S.	5.5	P<.001	27
2L	Kang et al,[24] 2016 GATSBY	345 (1:2)	Pac38%/Doc 62%	OS (No)	8.6	1.15	2.9	1.13	20
			T-DM1		7.9	P = N.S.	2.7	P = N.S	21

Abbreviations: Cis/FP, cisplatin + fluoropyrimidine; Doc, docetaxel; Pac, paclitaxel.
[a] mOS and HR for IHC2-3+ & FISH+ subset.

positive.[23] Patients received paclitaxel alone or in combination with lapatinib. Despite response rates of 27% versus 9%, no statistically significant PFS or OS benefit was demonstrated in the ITT population. Of note, when limiting the evaluation to only those patients with 3+ IHC expression, median survival improved to 14 months from 7.6 months in this subgroup ($P = .0176$), with progression-free survival of 5.6 versus 4.2 months, respectively ($P = .0101$).

Trastuzumab emtansine (T-DM1), an antibody drug conjugate that is approved in HER2 positive metastatic breast cancer, was also studied in the second-line Study of Trastuzumab Emtansine (T-DM1) Versus Taxane in Patients with Previously Treated HER2-Positive Locally Advanced or Metastatic GEC (GATSBY) trial for HER2 positive GEC (see **Table 2**), but this failed to support a response or survival benefit versus paclitaxel monotherapy.[24] Possible explanations for this negative trial include intrapatient HER2 tumor heterogeneity, which is more frequent in GEC than observed in breast cancer.[25] With clonal heterogeneity, it has been hypothesized that HER2 negative (or low expressing) clones are not controlled by HER2-targeted cytotoxic therapy. Furthermore, HER2 expression/amplification has been demonstrated to convert after first-line therapy. Archived specimen testing, as used in both second-line trials (GATSBY and TyTAN), may therefore lead to inadequate HER2 positive patient selection in subsequent line trials.[26–29] Specifically, a recent phase II randomized study of paclitaxel plus trastuzumab versus paclitaxel, trastuzumab plus MM-111 (a bivalent antibody toward HER2 and HER3) was conducted in the second-line setting after failure of first-line cytotoxic therapy for HER2 positive cancers. Trial enrollment eligibility was based upon archived original diagnostic samples, and correlative studies demonstrated this *HER2* amplification molecular evolution concern. In this trial, the median overall survival of 44 patients receiving trastuzumab and paclitaxel was 14 months versus 8 months in the 44 patients receiving MM-111, trastuzumab, and paclitaxel (HR 2.12, $P = .045$, 95% confidence interval [CI] 1.0–4.5). Interestingly, central HER2 testing of the 66% of available original archived samples revealed that 30% of cases were actually considered IHC 0/1+% and 8% IHC2 positive/FISH negative, demonstrating an overall 38% of cases that would never have been considered HER2 positive. This could be caused by a combination of factors including intratumoral HER2 heterogeneity testing different regions spatially within a tumor, or technique/assay variability and subjective scoring. Importantly, of approximately 40 patients having matched archival and fresh biopsy prior to initiating second-line therapy, approximately 15% of patients initially considered HER2 positive were later found to be HER2 negative prior to second-line therapy initiation. Regardless, approximately 50% of patients enrolled into this HER2 positive selection trial were considered HER2 negative in retrospect. Future trials evaluating the role of anti-HER2 therapy for GEC patients after failure of prior anti-HER2 therapy should therefore mandate fresh biopsy (and/or possibly cfDNA assessment) to confirm the presence of HER2 positivity at the time of enrollment and thereby ensure proper treatment arm stratification by HER2 status.

As alluded to previously, although HER-2 overexpression/*ERBB2* amplification predicts benefit from the anti-HER2 antibody trastuzumab in the first-line setting,[15,30] the definitions of positivity and trial inclusion criteria have evolved over time. Current clinical diagnostic testing requires evaluation by a combination of IHC (membranous reactivity in at least 10% of cancer cells in a surgical specimen or a cluster of at least 5 cells in a biopsy specimen) and fluorescence in situ hybridization (FISH with HER2:CEP17 ratio $\geq$2). IHC 0/1 is now considered negative, and IHC3 positive is considered positive, while IHC2 positive requires reflex to FISH assessment. Higher throughput assays, including mass spectrometry and next-generation sequencing (NGS), have emerged with the potential to refine diagnostic accuracy and allow multiplexing capability to assess for other relevant aberrations with limited tissue samples.[5,22,29] Similarly, circulating cell-free DNA (cfDNA) is emerging as a potential noninvasive method, particularly for serial *ERBB2* amplification,[31] which may provide further insight into tumor genetic evolution.[26–29]

Nevertheless, to date, no standard anti-HER2 directed approaches are recognized in trastuzumab-refractory HER2 positive GEC using any available diagnostic testing. Standard chemotherapy with irinotecan or taxane-based regimens is recommended. Notably, while second-line ramucirumab trials included HER2 positive and trastuzumab-treated patients, this accounted for only approximately 6% of patients enrolled in the Ramucirumab Montherapy for Previously Treated Advanced Gastric or Gastro-oesophageal Junction Adenocarcinoma (REGARD) trial and less than 1% of patients enrolled in the REGARD trial (Medical Letter).[32,33] Other strategies under evaluation in the second and later lines include novel TKIs like afatinib,[34] trastuzumab beyond progression (and ensuring persisting HER2 positivity),[26,27] novel HER2 antibodies,[35] and combination therapy with immune checkpoint inhibitors (NCT02689284).

Neoadjuvant HER2-directed therapy has been integrated into routine breast cancer therapy based on the phase III NeOAdjuvant Herceptin (NOAH) trial, which identified an improved 5-year event-free survival and overall survival with the addition of trastuzumab to neoadjuvant chemotherapy.[36] Similarly, the GeparQuattro trial demonstrated increased pathologic complete remission with neoadjuvant trastuzumab in HER2-positive breast cancer patients,[37] which was further increased by combining trastuzumab and lapatinib with chemotherapy in the NeoALTTO trial.[38] Based on these results and the ToGA trial,[17] RTOG1010 explores neoadjuvant chemoradiation in EGJ with carboplatin and paclitaxel with or without trastuzumab. Accrual has been completed, and results are awaited (NCT01196390). Similarly, the neoadjuvant Integration of Trastuzumab, With or Without Pertuzumab, into Perioperative Chemotherapy of HER-2 Positive Stomach Cancer (INNOVATION) trial is evaluating the addition of trastuzumab and pertuzumab to cisplatin and fluoropyrimidine doublet therapy in GEC.[39] The phase II HER-FLOT trial identified an R0 resection rate of 93.3% and pathologic complete remission in 22.2% of patients when trastuzumab was added to perioperative 5-FU, oxaliplatin, leucovorin, and docetaxel (FLOT).[40] A similar phase II study combining FOLFIRINOX and trastuzumab in the perioperative setting remains underway (NCT02782182). These findings will be further explored in the phase III FLOT vs FLOT/Herceptin/Pertuzumab for Perioperative Therapy of HER-2 Expressing Gastric or GEJ Cancer (PETRARCA) study, which randomizes patients to receive perioperative FLOT with or without trastuzumab and pertuzumab (NCT02581462). Until these results from these trials are available, however, HER2-targeted therapy is not considered standard of care for GEC in the neoadjuvant setting.

Epidermal Growth Factor Receptor

Epidermal growth factor receptor (EGFR) or ERBB1 is a transmembrane receptor and a well-recognized mediator of oncogenic phenotype that is expressed in approximately 30% of GECs.[41,42] EGFR-overexpressing tumors are associated with higher stage, more poorly differentiated histology, increased vascular invasion, and potentially shorter survival.[13,43] *EGFR* amplification and consequent overexpression is found in only 2% to 6% of GEC patients, and mutations in less than 2%, although the functional and therapeutic implications of these aberrations are yet to be clearly defined (see **Table 1**).[9,44,45]

EGFR-directed therapies include monoclonal antibodies such as cetuximab and panitumumab, which antagonize the extracellular binding domain. Preclinical data also suggests that cetuximab, a recombinant human–murine chimeric monoclonal antibody of a murine Fv region and a human immunoglobulin (Ig)G1 heavy and k light chain Fc region, also induces ADCC similar to trastuzumab.[46] Small molecule TKIs, such as gefitinib, erlotinib, lapatinib, and afatinib competitively bind intracellularly to the tyrosine kinase domain at varying potencies and specificities. Early phase II trials combining cetuximab, panitumumab, or erlotinib with cytotoxic chemotherapy in unselected GEC patients identified first-line therapy response rates from 41% to 65%.[47–50] Second-line phase II evaluations of gefitinib or erlotinib monotherapy led to more modest responses of approximately 9% to 11%, and responses appeared higher in proximal EGJ cancers rather than distal GC.[51,52]

Subsequent phase III GEC trials targeting EGFR included Erbitux in Combination With Xeloda and Cisplatin in Advanced Esophagogastric Cancer (EXPAND) (cetuximab plus capecitabin/cisplatin, first line), Randomised ECF for Advanced or Locally advanced oesophagogastric cancer-3 (REAL-3) (panitumumab plus epirubicin/oxaliplatin/capecitabine, first line), and Cancer Oesophagus Gefitinib (COG) (gefitinib monotherapy, second line) (**Table 3**).[53–55] Disappointingly, each trial was resoundingly negative, and panitumumab actually resulted in worse survival compared with the control. Notably, each of these trials enrolled all comers without biomarker selection of any kind.

Preclinically, 20% of patient-derived xenografts responded to cetuximab, and of these responders, half were later found to harbor *EGFR* amplification.[56] In the phase II study combining FOLFOX with cetuximab, 22% of patients had more than 4 *EGFR* copies, which correlated with increased overall survival.[57] Similarly, in TRANS-COG, the preplanned translational correlative study of COG, 15.6% of patients had increased gene copy number (GCN) including true *EGFR* amplification (ratio *EGFR/ CEP7* $\geq$2) ($\sim$5%); this latter small subset of *EGFR* amplified patients derived a statistically significant survival benefit with the addition of gefitinib (HR 0.19, P = .007).[58] The EXPAND trial also demonstrated survival benefit in the small subset with extremely high EGFR expression by IHC H-Score (likely representing EGFR amplified tumors, but yet to be confirmed).[59] Thus, with these recent promising subset analyses of *EGFR* amplification and consequent overexpression, future studies assessing the benefits of anti-EGFR therapy in these patients are being pursued.[60] A phase III trial of second-line nimotuzumab with irinotecan (NCT01813253) is also currently recruiting patients deemed to harbor EGFR overexpressing (IHC 2/3+) tumors.

MET

The MET protooncogene encodes the c-MET receptor tyrosine kinase, which is involved in cell proliferation, angiogenesis, and migration. MET overexpressing and *MET* amplified tumors are each associated with worse survival.[43,44,61–69] Canonical MET activation occurs via binding of its ligand, hepatocyte growth factor (HGF), but MET activation can also occur in an HGF-independent manner through RTK cross-talk (see **Fig. 1**).[70,71] *MET* amplification leads to constitutive receptor activation independent of ligand, and is reported in approximately 4 to 10% of GEC cases,[44,72–74] but overexpression ranges from 25% to 70% by IHC in GEC (see **Table 1**).[64–66,75–77]

Early phase reports and trials suggested that MET expression may serve as a predictive biomarker for MET-directed therapeutic response in GEC patients.[69,75] A subsequent phase II,[78] and 2 phase III MET-directed trials in GEC, however, have all reported overall negative results (**Table 4**).[79,80] The first-line METGastric phase III study evaluated onartuzumab, a humanized IgG1 antibody against the extracellular domain of c-MET, in combination with mFOLFOX6, in patients with c-MET-expressing tumors ($\geq$1+, $\geq$50% cells).[80] However, METGastric was terminated prematurely (70% of planned accrual) because of negative results (in any predefined MET expression subgroup) reported from the prior/parallel YO28252 phase II biomarker evaluation trial of onartuzumab enrolling unselected GEC patients.[78] With this in mind, no benefit was seen in the METGastric ITT, nor in the MET IHC 2-3 positive preplanned subgroup

Table 3
Epidemial growth factor receptor-directed phase III clinical trials for gastroesophageal cancer

Line	Trial	N	Treatment	1° Endpt (Met?)	mOS (mo)	HR	mPFS (mo)	HR	RR (%)
1L	Lordick et al,[53] 2014 EXPAND	904	Cis/Cape/placebo Cis/Cape/cetuximab	PFS (No)	10.7 9.4	1.00	5.6 4.4	1.09 $P = .32$	29 30
1L	Wadcell et al,[54] 2013 REAL-3	553	Epi/Oxali/Cape-Pl Epi/Oxali/Cape-P	OS (No)	11.3 8.8	1.37 $P = .013$	7.4 6.0	1.22	42 46
2L	Dutton et al,[55] 2014 COG	450	Placebo Gefitinib	OS (No)	3.67 3.73	0.9	1.17 1.57	0.8	~1 ~4

Abbreviations: Cis/Cape, cisplatin/capecitabine; Epi/Oxali/Cape, epirubicin/oxaliplatin/capecitabine; Pl, placebo; P, panitumumab.

Table 4
MET-directed phase II/III clinical trials for gastroesophageal cancer

Line	Trial	N	Treatment	1° Endpoint (Met?)	mOS (mo)	HR	mPFS (mo)	HR	RR (%)
1L	Cunningham et al,[79] 2015 RILOMET-1	609	Epi/Cis/5FU/placebo	OS (No)	11.5	1.37	5.7	1.3	39
			Epi/Cis/5FU/rilotumumab		9.6	P = .016	5.7		30
1L	Shah et al,[80] 2015 MET-GASTRIC	562	FOLFOX/placebo	OS (No)	11.3	0.82	6.8	0.9	41
			FOLFOX-onartuzumab		11	P = .24	6.7		46
1L	Shah et al,[78] 2016 YO28252	123	FOLFOX6/placebo	PFS (No)	11.27	1.06	6.97	1.08	57.1
			FOLFOX6-onartuzumab		10.61	P = .83	6.77	0.71	60.5

Abbreviation: Epi/Cis/5FU, epirubicin/cisplatin/5-fluorouracil.

analysis (which accounted for ~38% of enrolled patients, HR 0.64, $P = .06$); this subgroup notably now possessed less power to identify a true benefit due to early termination of the trial.[80] Similarly, Rilotumumab With Cisplatin and Capecitabine (CX) as First-line Therapy in Advanced MET-Positive Gastric or Gastroesophageal Junction Adenocarcinoma (RILOMET-1), evaluated first-line epirubicin, cisplatin, and capecitabine (ECX) with or without the addition of rilotumomab, a fully human IgG2 antibody against HGF ligand, for MET-expressing GEC was terminated because of an increased risk of death from the study drug.[79]

One pitfall of these phase III trials was their loose definition of MET expression. In RILOMET-1, trial inclusion required at least 1+ MET expression by IHC in at least 25% of tumor cells, accounting for 81% of patients screened. Of all patients enrolled, only 21% of tumors had high expression ($\geq$2+, $\geq$50% cells). Similarly, only 38% of METGastric patients were IHC 2-3 positive in at least 50% of cells, yet previously described, these patients demonstrated a near-significant benefit, in an underaccrued trial. Thus, even with the large phase III MET inhibitor trials, one could argue that the selection for MET-dependent cancers was overly lenient, and the highest expressing tumors clearly under-represented, particularly in RILOMET-1.[44,72-74]

More promising results, however, have been reported in smaller earlier phase trials of MET inhibitors in MET-amplified patients (4%–5% of GEC),[44,65,72,74] with consequent over-expression.[72] AMG-337, a relatively highly selective MET TKI, demonstrated clinical responses in MET-amplified advanced GEC patients (ORR 50%), but the phase II expansion phase of the trial has been on hold (results not publically available).[81] Similarly, half of MET-amplified patients treated with crizotinib in a phase I expansion cohort-experienced response,[82] and 75% of MET-amplified patients receiving ABT-700 monoclonal antibody monotherapy demonstrated an objective response.[82] The challenge of molecular heterogeneity,[26,83] particularly in the CIN subset of GEC,[9] may account for lack of response and/or rapid development of resistance to MET-directed monotherapy of MET-amplified GEC. Any future therapeutic attempts of the MET pathway will likely be directed toward the small MET-amplified subset of patients,[84] in conjunction with cytotoxic agents,[52] other targeted therapies, and/or immune checkpoint inhibitors either in combination or in sequential fashion to achieve optimal benefit.

SUMMARY

Development of molecularly targeted therapies in GEC has been hindered by inadequate predictive biomarkers. With respect to HER2, despite the breast cancer and ToGA experiences, patients with HER2 FISH positive but IHC negative disease were included in the Tytan (36% of patients) and LOGiC (17% of patients) trials.[19,23] Moreover, 10.4% of patients in the GATSBY trial harbored IHC3 positive/FISH negative tumors compared with the ToGA trial's 2.3%, raising the question as to whether this IHC3 positive/FISH negative molecular subset should be considered similar or dissimilar to the IHC3 positive/FISH positive genomic driver subset. Furthermore, nearly one-third of cases in the second-line trastuzumab with/without MM-111 were later reclassified as HER2 negative, and another 15% were no longer HER2 positive upon repeat biopsy after first-line progression, suggesting that updated HER2 testing prior to each line might be necessary for optimal patient selection.[27] For MET, although early trials suggested MET expression as a predictive biomarker for anti-MET therapies, the RILOMET-1 trial MET expression requirements may have been too loose, and the power for METGastric to identify a more likely HR of approximately 0.7 to 0.8 was low given that the trial was underaccrued because of early termination.[79] Finally, in the phase III EGFR trials, no biomarkers of selection were utilized. All of the evidence suggests that targeted therapies may have a role, but in more targeted select patient populations. Finally, using alternative diagnostic platforms, including DNA amplification and mass spectroscopy, it may be feasible to better select the appropriate patient population in future studies.[60]

Although approximately one-third to one-half of patients with GEC harbor potentially actionable alterations, patient population selection with varying scoring, heterogeneity, and/or infrequent incidence has stifled clinical trial success. As of 2016, only trastuzumab has been approved for first-line GEC patients in a select HER2-positive population. Subset analyses have identified patients with *MET* and *EGFR* amplifications that are more likely to benefit from respective targeted therapies, albeit for a finite period of time before various developed resistance mechanisms emerge. Intrapatient molecular heterogeneity is also emerging as a considerable hurdle for targeted therapies.[26] However, designing traditional trials for such infrequent genomic aberrations remains difficult. One solution may be further development of novel trial designs such as the personalized anti-neoplastics for gastroesophageal adenocarcinoma (PANGEA) type II expansion platform trial (particularly with serial assessment and 're-targeting' over time) that may better identify and treat these uncommon actionable aberrations by testing an overall treatment strategy composed of various biomarker/drug pairings, and compare this personalized treatment strategy outcome to a treatment control arm.[60]

REFERENCES

1. Torre LA, Bray F, Siegel RL, et al. Global cancer statistics, 2012. CA Cancer J Clin 2015;65(2):87–108.
2. Sehdev A, Catenacci DV. Gastroesophageal cancer: focus on epidemiology, classification, and staging. Discov Med 2013;16(87):103–11.
3. Sehdev A, Catenacci DV. Perioperative therapy for locally advanced gastroesophageal cancer: current controversies and consensus of care. J Hematol Oncol 2013;6:66.
4. Siegel RL, Miller KD, Jemal A. Cancer statistics, 2015. CA Cancer J Clin 2015; 65(1):5–29.
5. Ali SM, Sanford EM, Klempner SJ, et al. Prospective comprehensive genomic profiling of advanced gastric carcinoma cases reveals frequent clinically relevant genomic alterations and new routes for targeted therapies. Oncologist 2015; 20(5):499–507.
6. Deng N, Goh LK, Wang H, et al. A comprehensive survey of genomic alterations in gastric cancer reveals systematic patterns of molecular exclusivity and co-occurrence among distinct therapeutic targets. Gut 2012;61(5):673–84.
7. Stachler MD, Taylor-Weiner A, Peng S, et al. Paired exome analysis of Barrett's esophagus and adenocarcinoma. Nat Genet 2015;47(9):1047–55.
8. Zang ZJ, Ong CK, Cutcutache I, et al. Genetic and structural variation in the gastric cancer kinome revealed through targeted deep sequencing. Cancer Res 2011;71(1):29–39.
9. Cancer Genome Atlas Research Network. Comprehensive molecular characterization of gastric adenocarcinoma. Nature 2014;513(7517):202–9.
10. Kameda T, Yasui W, Yoshida K, et al. Expression of ERBB2 in human gastric carcinomas: relationship between p185ERBB2 expression and the gene amplification. Cancer Res 1990;50(24):8002–9.
11. Okines AF, Thompson LC, Cunningham D, et al. Effect of HER2 on prognosis and benefit from peri-operative chemotherapy in early oesophago-gastric adenocarcinoma in the MAGIC trial. Ann Oncol 2013;24(5):1253–61.

12. Gordon MA, Gundacker HM, Benedetti J, et al. Assessment of HER2 gene amplification in adenocarcinomas of the stomach or gastroesophageal junction in the INT-0116/SWOG9008 clinical trial. Ann Oncol 2013;24(7):1754–61.
13. Terashima M, Kitada K, Ochiai A, et al. Impact of expression of human epidermal growth factor receptors EGFR and ERBB2 on survival in stage II/III gastric cancer. Clin Cancer Res 2012;18(21):5992–6000.
14. Kurokawa Y, Matsuura N, Kimura Y, et al. Multicenter large-scale study of prognostic impact of HER2 expression in patients with resectable gastric cancer. Gastric Cancer 2015;18(4):691–7.
15. Bang YJ, Van Cutsem E, Feyereislova A, et al. Trastuzumab in combination with chemotherapy versus chemotherapy alone for treatment of HER2-positive advanced gastric or gastro-oesophageal junction cancer (ToGA): a phase 3, open-label, randomised controlled trial. Lancet 2010;376(9742):687–97.
16. Hofmann M, Stoss O, Shi D, et al. Assessment of a HER2 scoring system for gastric cancer: results from a validation study. Histopathology 2008;52(7): 797–805.
17. Swain SM, Kim SB, Cortes J, et al. Pertuzumab, trastuzumab, and docetaxel for HER2-positive metastatic breast cancer (CLEOPATRA study): overall survival results from a randomised, double-blind, placebo-controlled, phase 3 study. Lancet Oncol 2013;14(6):461–71.
18. Tabernero J, Hoff PM, Shen L, et al. Pertuzumab (P) with trastuzumab (T) and chemotherapy (CTX) in patients (pts) with HER2-positive metastatic gastric or gastroesophageal junction (GEJ) cancer: an international phase III study (JACOB). Paper presented at: ASCO Annual Meeting Proceedings. Chicago, June 2, 2013.
19. Hecht JR, Bang YJ, Qin SK, et al. Lapatinib in combination with capecitabine plus oxaliplatin in human epidermal growth factor receptor 2-positive advanced or metastatic gastric, esophageal, or gastroesophageal adenocarcinoma: TRIO-013/LOGiC–a randomized phase III trial. J Clin Oncol 2016;34(5):443–51.
20. Gomez-Martin C, Plaza JC, Pazo-Cid R, et al. Level of HER2 gene amplification predicts response and overall survival in HER2-positive advanced gastric cancer treated with trastuzumab. J Clin Oncol 2013;31(35):4445–52.
21. Ock CY, Lee KW, Kim JW, et al. Optimal patient selection for trastuzumab treatment in HER2-positive advanced gastric cancer. Clin Cancer Res 2015;21(11):2520–9.
22. Catenacci DV, Liao WL, Zhao L, et al. Mass-spectrometry-based quantitation of Her2 in gastroesophageal tumor tissue: comparison to IHC and FISH. Gastric Cancer 2016;19(4):1066–79.
23. Satoh T, Xu RH, Chung HC, et al. Lapatinib plus paclitaxel versus paclitaxel alone in the second-line treatment of HER2-amplified advanced gastric cancer in Asian populations: TyTAN–a randomized, phase III study. J Clin Oncol 2014;32(19): 2039–49.
24. Kang Y-K, Shah MA, Ohtsu A, et al. A randomized, open-label, multicenter, adaptive phase 2/3 study of trastuzumab emtansine (T-DM1) versus a taxane (TAX) in patients (pts) with previously treated HER2-positive locally advanced or metastatic gastric/gastroesophageal junction adenocarcinoma (LA/MGC/GEJC). Paper presented at: ASCO Annual Meeting Proceedings. Chicago, June 5, 2013.
25. Yang J, Luo H, Li Y, et al. Intratumoral heterogeneity determines discordant results of diagnostic tests for human epidermal growth factor receptor (HER) 2 in gastric cancer specimens. Cell Biochem Biophys 2012;62(1):221–8.
26. Catenacci DV. Next-generation clinical trials: Novel strategies to address the challenge of tumor molecular heterogeneity. Mol Oncol 2015;9(5):967–96.

27. Denlinger CS, Alsina Maqueda M, Watkins DJ, et al. Randomized phase 2 study of paclitaxel (PTX), trastuzumab (T) with or without MM-111 in HER2 expressing gastroesophageal cancers (GEC). Paper presented at: ASCO Annual Meeting Proceedings. Chicago, June 5, 2013.

28. Janjigian YY, Riches JC, Ku GY, et al. Loss of human epidermal growth factor receptor 2 (HER2) expression in HER2-overexpressing esophagogastric (EG) tumors treated with trastuzumab. Paper presented at: ASCO Annual Meeting Proceedings. Chicago, May 31, 2015.

29. Sellappan S, Blackler A, Liao WL, et al. Therapeutically induced changes in HER2, HER3, and EGFR protein expression for treatment guidance. J Natl Compr Canc Netw 2016;14(5):503–7.

30. Hofmann M, Stoss O, Gaiser T, et al. Central HER2 IHC and FISH analysis in a trastuzumab (Herceptin) phase II monotherapy study: assessment of test sensitivity and impact of chromosome 17 polysomy. J Clin Pathol 2008;61(1):89–94.

31. Shoda K, Masuda K, Ichikawa D, et al. HER2 amplification detected in the circulating DNA of patients with gastric cancer: a retrospective pilot study. Gastric Cancer 2015;18(4):698–710.

32. Wilke H, Muro K, Van Cutsem E, et al. Ramucirumab plus paclitaxel versus placebo plus paclitaxel in patients with previously treated advanced gastric or gastro-oesophageal junction adenocarcinoma (RAINBOW): a double-blind, randomised phase 3 trial. Lancet Oncol 2014;15(11):1224–35.

33. Fuchs CS, Tomasek J, Yong CJ, et al. Ramucirumab monotherapy for previously treated advanced gastric or gastro-oesophageal junction adenocarcinoma (REGARD): an international, randomised, multicentre, placebo-controlled, phase 3 trial. Lancet 2014;383(9911):31–9.

34. Janjigian YY, Capanu M, Imtiaz T, et al. A phase II study of afatinib in patients (pts) with metastatic human epidermal growth factor receptor (HER2)-positive trastuzumab-refractory esophagogastric (EG) cancer. Paper presented at: ASCO Annual Meeting Proceedings. Chicago, June 1, 2014.

35. Rugo HS, Pegram MD, Gradishar WJ, et al. SOPHIA: A phase 3, randomized study of margetuximab (M) plus chemotherapy (CTX) vs trastuzumab (T) plus CTX in the treatment of patients with HER2+ metastatic breast cancer (MBC). ASCO Meet Abstr 2016;34(15_suppl):TPS630.

36. Gianni L, Eiermann W, Semiglazov V, et al. Neoadjuvant and adjuvant trastuzumab in patients with HER2-positive locally advanced breast cancer (NOAH): follow-up of a randomised controlled superiority trial with a parallel HER2-negative cohort. Lancet Oncol 2014;15(6):640–7.

37. Untch M, Rezai M, Loibl S, et al. Neoadjuvant treatment with trastuzumab in HER2-positive breast cancer: results from the GeparQuattro study. J Clin Oncol 2010;28(12):2024–31.

38. Baselga J, Bradbury I, Eidtmann H, et al. Lapatinib with trastuzumab for HER2-positive early breast cancer (NeoALTTO): a randomised, open-label, multicentre, phase 3 trial. Lancet 2012;379(9816):633–40.

39. Wagner AD, Kang Y-K, van Dieren J, et al. EORTC-1203: Integration of trastuzumab (T), with or without pertuzumab (P), into perioperative chemotherapy (CT) of HER-2 positive stomach cancer–INNOVATION trial. ASCO Meet Abstr 2016; 34(15_suppl):TPS4133.

40. Hofheinz R, Hegewisch-Becker S, Thuss-Patience PC, et al. HER-FLOT: Trastuzumab in combination with FLOT as perioperative treatment for patients with HER2-positive locally advanced esophagogastric adenocarcinoma: a phase II trial of

the AIO Gastric Cancer Study Group. Paper presented at: ASCO Annual Meeting Proceedings. Chicago, June 1, 2014.

41. Kim MA, Lee HS, Lee HE, et al. EGFR in gastric carcinomas: prognostic significance of protein overexpression and high gene copy number. Histopathology 2008;52(6):738–46.

42. Wang KL, Wu TT, Choi IS, et al. Expression of epidermal growth factor receptor in esophageal and esophagogastric junction adenocarcinomas: association with poor outcome. Cancer 2007;109(4):658–67.

43. Nagatsuma AK, Aizawa M, Kuwata T, et al. Expression profiles of HER2, EGFR, MET and FGFR2 in a large cohort of patients with gastric adenocarcinoma. Gastric Cancer 2015;18(2):227–38.

44. Lennerz JK, Kwak EL, Ackerman A, et al. MET amplification identifies a small and aggressive subgroup of esophagogastric adenocarcinoma with evidence of responsiveness to crizotinib. J Clin Oncol 2011;29(36):4803–10.

45. Dulak AM, Stojanov P, Peng S, et al. Exome and whole-genome sequencing of esophageal adenocarcinoma identifies recurrent driver events and mutational complexity. Nat Genet 2013;45(5):478–86.

46. Kimura H, Sakai K, Arao T, et al. Antibody-dependent cellular cytotoxicity of cetuximab against tumor cells with wild-type or mutant epidermal growth factor receptor. Cancer Sci 2007;98(8):1275–80.

47. Enzinger PC, Burtness BA, Niedzwiecki D, et al. CALGB 80403 (Alliance)/E1206: a randomized phase II study of three chemotherapy regimens plus cetuximab in metastatic esophageal and gastroesophageal junction cancers. J Clin Oncol 2016;34(23):2736–42.

48. Wainberg ZA, Lin LS, DiCarlo B, et al. Phase II trial of modified FOLFOX6 and erlotinib in patients with metastatic or advanced adenocarcinoma of the oesophagus and gastro-oesophageal junction. Br J Cancer 2011;105(6):760–5.

49. Lordick F, Luber B, Lorenzen S, et al. Cetuximab plus oxaliplatin/leucovorin/5-fluorouracil in first-line metastatic gastric cancer: a phase II study of the Arbeitsgemeinschaft Internistische Onkologie (AIO). Br J Cancer 2010;102(3):500–5.

50. Tebbutt NC, Price TJ, Ferraro DA, et al. Panitumumab added to docetaxel, cisplatin and fluoropyrimidine in oesophagogastric cancer: ATTAX3 phase II trial. Br J Cancer 2016;114(5):505–9.

51. Ferry DR, Anderson M, Beddard K, et al. A phase II study of gefitinib monotherapy in advanced esophageal adenocarcinoma: evidence of gene expression, cellular, and clinical response. Clin Cancer Res 2007;13(19):5869–75.

52. Dragovich T, McCoy S, Fenoglio-Preiser CM, et al. Phase II trial of erlotinib in gastroesophageal junction and gastric adenocarcinomas: SWOG 0127. J Clin Oncol 2006;24(30):4922–7.

53. Lordick F, Kang YK, Chung HC, et al. Capecitabine and cisplatin with or without cetuximab for patients with previously untreated advanced gastric cancer (EXPAND): a randomised, open-label phase 3 trial. Lancet Oncol 2013;14(6):490–9.

54. Waddell T, Chau I, Cunningham D, et al. Epirubicin, oxaliplatin, and capecitabine with or without panitumumab for patients with previously untreated advanced oesophagogastric cancer (REAL3): a randomised, open-label phase 3 trial. Lancet Oncol 2013;14(6):481–9.

55. Dutton SJ, Ferry DR, Blazeby JM, et al. Gefitinib for oesophageal cancer progressing after chemotherapy (COG): a phase 3, multicentre, double-blind, placebo-controlled randomised trial. Lancet Oncol 2014;15(8):894–904.

56. Zhang L, Yang J, Cai J, et al. A subset of gastric cancers with EGFR amplification and overexpression respond to cetuximab therapy. Sci Rep 2013;3:2992.

57. Luber B, Deplazes J, Keller G, et al. Biomarker analysis of cetuximab plus oxaliplatin/leucovorin/5-fluorouracil in first-line metastatic gastric and oesophago-gastric junction cancer: results from a phase II trial of the Arbeitsgemeinschaft Internistische Onkologie (AIO). BMC Cancer 2011;11:509.

58. Petty RD, Dahle-Smith A, Miedzybrodzka Z, et al. Epidermal growth factor receptor copy number gain (EGFR CNG) and response to gefitinib in esophageal cancer (EC): Results of a biomarker analysis of a phase III trial of gefitinib versus placebo (TRANS-COG). J Clin Oncol (Meeting Abstracts) 2014;32(15_suppl): 4016.

59. Lordick F, Kang Y-K, Salman P, et al. Clinical outcome according to tumor HER2 status and EGFR expression in advanced gastric cancer patients from the EXPAND study. Paper presented at: ASCO Annual Meeting Proceedings. Chicago, June 2, 2013.

60. Catenacci DVT, Polite BN, Henderson L, et al. Toward personalized treatment for gastroesophageal adenocarcinoma (GEC): Strategies to address tumor heterogeneity–PANGEA. Paper presented at: ASCO Annual Meeting Proceedings. Chicago, June 1, 2014.

61. Catenacci DVT, Tang R, Oliner KS, et al. MET as a prognostic biomarker of survival in a large cohort of patients with gastroesophageal cancer (GEC). Paper presented at: ASCO Annual Meeting Proceedings. Chicago, May 31, 2015.

62. Hack SP, Bruey JM, Koeppen H. HGF/MET-directed therapeutics in gastroesophageal cancer: a review of clinical and biomarker development. Oncotarget 2014; 5(10):2866–80.

63. Metzger ML, Behrens HM, Boger C, et al. MET in gastric cancer–discarding a 10% cutoff rule. Histopathology 2016;68(2):241–53.

64. Nakajima M, Sawada H, Yamada Y, et al. The prognostic significance of amplification and overexpression of c-met and c-erb B-2 in human gastric carcinomas. Cancer 1999;85(9):1894–902.

65. Lee HE, Kim MA, Lee HS, et al. MET in gastric carcinomas: comparison between protein expression and gene copy number and impact on clinical outcome. Br J Cancer 2012;107(2):325–33.

66. Graziano F, Galluccio N, Lorenzini P, et al. Genetic activation of the MET pathway and prognosis of patients with high-risk, radically resected gastric cancer. J Clin Oncol 2011;29(36):4789–95.

67. Catenacci DV, Cervantes G, Yala S, et al. RON (MST1R) is a novel prognostic marker and therapeutic target for gastroesophageal adenocarcinoma. Cancer Biol Ther 2011;12(1):9–46.

68. Yu S, Yu Y, Zhao N, et al. C-Met as a prognostic marker in gastric cancer: a systematic review and meta-analysis. PLoS One 2013;8(11):e79137.

69. Iveson T, Donehower RC, Davidenko I, et al. Rilotumumab in combination with epirubicin, cisplatin, and capecitabine as first-line treatment for gastric or oesophagogastric junction adenocarcinoma: an open-label, dose de-escalation phase 1b study and a double-blind, randomised phase 2 study. Lancet Oncol 2014;15(9): 1007–18.

70. Jo M, Stolz DB, Esplen JE, et al. Cross-talk between epidermal growth factor receptor and c-Met signal pathways in transformed cells. J Biol Chem 2000; 275(12):8806–11.

71. Yamaguchi H, Chang SS, Hsu JL, et al. Signaling cross-talk in the resistance to HER family receptor targeted therapy. Oncogene 2014;33(9):1073–81.

72. Catenacci DV, Liao WL, Thyparambil S, et al. Absolute quantitation of Met using mass spectrometry for clinical application: assay precision, stability, and

correlation with MET gene amplification in FFPE tumor tissue. PLoS One 2014; 9(7):e100586.

73. Jardim DL, Tang C, Gagliato Dde M, et al. Analysis of 1,115 patients tested for MET amplification and therapy response in the MD Anderson phase I clinic. Clin Cancer Res 2014;20(24):6336–45.

74. Smolen GA, Sordella R, Muir B, et al. Amplification of MET may identify a subset of cancers with extreme sensitivity to the selective tyrosine kinase inhibitor PHA-665752. Proc Natl Acad Sci U S A 2006;103(7):2316–21.

75. Catenacci DV, Henderson L, Xiao SY, et al. Durable complete response of metastatic gastric cancer with anti-Met therapy followed by resistance at recurrence. Cancer Discov 2011;1(7):573–9.

76. Toiyama Y, Yasuda H, Saigusa S, et al. Co-expression of hepatocyte growth factor and c-Met predicts peritoneal dissemination established by autocrine hepatocyte growth factor/c-Met signaling in gastric cancer. Int J Cancer 2012;130(12): 2912–21.

77. Zhao J, Zhang X, Xin Y. Up-regulated expression of Ezrin and c-Met proteins are related to the metastasis and prognosis of gastric carcinomas. Histol Histopathol 2011;26(9):1111–20.

78. Shah MA, Cho JY, Tan IB, et al. A Randomized Phase II Study of FOLFOX With or Without the MET inhibitor onartuzumab in advanced adenocarcinoma of the stomach and gastroesophageal junction. Oncologist 2016;21(9):1085–90.

79. Cunningham D. Phase III, randomized, double-blind, multicenter, placebo (P)-controlled trial of rilotumumab (R) plus epirubicin, cisplatin and capecitabine (ECX) as first-line therapy in patients (pts) with advanced MET-positive (pos) gastric or gastroesophageal junction (G/GEJ) cancer: RILOMET-1 study. J Clin Oncol 2015;33(Suppl).

80. Shah MA, Bang YJ, Lordick F, et al. Effect of fluorouracil, leucovorin, and oxaliplatin with or without onartuzumab in HER2-negative, MET-positive gastroesophageal adenocarcinoma: The METGastric randomized clinical trial. JAMA Oncol 2016.

81. Kwak EL, LoRusso P, Hamid O, et al. Clinical activity of AMG 337, an oral MET kinase inhibitor, in adult patients (pts) with MET-amplified gastroesophageal junction (GEJ), gastric (G), or esophageal (E) cancer. Paper presented at: ASCO Annual Meeting Proceedings. Chicago, May 31, 2015.

82. Kang Y-K, LoRusso P, Salgia R, et al. Phase I study of ABT-700, an anti-c-Met antibody, in patients (pts) with advanced gastric or esophageal cancer (GEC). Paper presented at: ASCO Annual Meeting Proceedings. Chicago, May 31, 2015.

83. Kwak EL, Ahronian LG, Siravegna G, et al. Molecular heterogeneity and receptor coamplification drive resistance to targeted therapy in MET-amplified esophagogastric cancer. Cancer Discov 2015;5(12):1271–81.

84. Mullard A. NCI-MATCH trial pushes cancer umbrella trial paradigm. Nat Rev Drug Discov 2015;14(8):513–5.

85. Van Cutsem E, Bang YJ, Feng-Yi F, et al. HER2 screening data from ToGA: targeting HER2 in gastric and gastroesophageal junction cancer. Gastric Cancer 2015; 18(3):476–84.

Emerging Novel Therapeutic Agents in the Treatment of Patients with Gastroesophageal and Gastric Adenocarcinoma

Gayathri Anandappa, MBBS, MRCP(UK), MPhil(Cantab)[a,b],
Ian Chau, MBBS, FRCP(UK), MD[a,b,*]

KEYWORDS

- Gastric adenocarcinoma • Gastroesophageal adenocarcinoma • FGFR2 inhibitors
- Claudin inhibitors • STAT3 inhibitors • MMP inhibitors • AZD4547 • Napabucasin

KEY POINTS

- With further understanding of the biology of gastric and gastroesophageal adenocarcinomas (GC), strides are being made to find effective treatments through novel trial designs.
- This article focuses on the ongoing trials of drugs targeting specific hallmarks of gastric and gastroesophageal cancers, including oncogene addiction proliferative pathways (fibroblast growth factor receptor 2 amplified tumors), stem cell inhibition, apoptotic induction through claudin inhibitors, and matrix metalloproteinase inhibition.
- In developing novel therapeutics in treatment of patients with GC, it is clear that parallel research efforts to refine target population and biomarkers are crucial, and targeting the tumor genomics and microenvironment may be key in improving overall survival.

INTRODUCTION

Gastric and gastroesophageal cancers (GC) are the third leading cause of cancer-related death world-wide with a combined incidence of nearly 1.4 million cases diagnosed annually.[1] Although the incidence of GC has decreased in most parts of the

Conflict of Interests: I. Chau is on the Advisory Board of Sanofi Oncology, Eli-Lilly, Bristol Meyers Squibb, MSD, Merck Serono, Gilead Science, Bayer, Novartis, and Macrogenics; has received research funding from Janssen-Cilag, Sanofi Oncology, Roche, Merck-Serono, and Novartis; and has received honorarium from Taiho, Pfizer, Amgen, Eli-Lilly, and Bayer. G. Anandappa declares no competing interests.
[a] Department of Medicine, The Royal Marsden Hospital NHS Foundation Trust, Downs Road, Sutton, Surrey SM2 5PT, UK; [b] Department of Medicine, Royal Marsden Hospital, London, UK
* Corresponding author. Department of Medicine, Royal Marsden Hospital, Downs Road, Sutton, Surrey SM2 5PT, UK.
E-mail address: ian.chau@rmh.nhs.uk

Hematol Oncol Clin N Am 31 (2017) 529–544
http://dx.doi.org/10.1016/j.hoc.2017.02.001
0889-8588/17/© 2017 Elsevier Inc. All rights reserved.

world, overall survival (OS) rates remain poor in patients with advanced disease. The challenges of achieving durable responses have been the marked heterogeneity in GCs as with most solid tumors. The initiation and evolution of GC is a multistep process occurring on a background of varying degrees of genetic instability in combination with inflammation. GCs show all the well-described hallmarks of cancer[2] including sustained proliferative signaling, evasion of growth suppressors, resistance of apoptosis, enabling of replicative immortality, induction of angiogenesis, activation of invasion and metastasis, reprogramming of energy metabolism, evasion of immune destruction, and recruitment of normal cells to create a tumor microenvironment. Targeting growth signaling by oncogenes including *HER2*, *EGFR*, and *MET*, antiangiogenic strategies, and checkpoint inhibition using immunotherapy are discussed elsewhere in this issue. This article focuses on drugs currently in clinical trials targeting other pathways including oncogene addiction proliferation pathways (fibroblast growth factor [FGF] 2 receptor [FGFR] amplified tumors), novel stem cell inhibitors of replicative immortality (signal transducers and activators of transcription [STAT] 3 inhibitors), induction of apoptosis by antibody and complement mediated cytotoxicity (CLDN18.2 inhibitors), and prevention of invasion and metastases (matrix metalloproteinase [MMP] inhibitors).

FIBROBLAST GROWTH FACTOR RECEPTOR 2 INHIBITORS

FGF and FGFR are a ubiquitous family involved in tissue repair, hematopoiesis, angiogenesis, and embryonic development. There are 18 ligands and four receptors through which the FGF signal (FGFR1-4); ligand binding results in FGFR dimerization, autophosphorylation, and signaling through PI3K-AKT or mitogen-activated protein kinase (MAPK) pathways. Dysregulation of FGFR signaling can occur because of receptor overexpression, gene amplification, mutation, or aberrant transcriptional regulation, and has been described in multiple cancers, including gastric cancers.[3–5] FGFR2 overexpression has been described in 30% to 40% of gastric cancers by immunohistochemistry[6] and FGFR2 amplification by polymerase chain reaction–based copy number assay was detected in 3% to 10% of gastric adenocarcinomas[7] and more recently by circulating DNA.[8]

FGFR2 amplification is associated with poor prognosis in patients with gastric cancer. In a study where amplification (5%–10%) and polysomy (>20%) of FGFR2 was identified by fluorescent in situ hybridization (FISH) assay in 961 patients with gastric cancer from United Kingdom, China, and Korea, the clinicopathologic and OS data suggested that FGFR2 amplification was associated with increased lymph node metastasis and poor OS. In the Korean cohort OS was 1.83 years compared with 6.17 years ($P = .0073$) without the amplification; in the UK cohort the OS was 0.45 compared with 1.9 years ($P = .0002$).[9] Multiple FGFR2 inhibitors have been developed and are in the phase 2 drug development pipeline.

AZD4547

AZD4547 is an oral, highly selective, potent ATP- competitive, small molecule tyrosine kinase inhibitor of FGFR1, 2, and 3. Its effects were tested in gastric cancer cell lines with FGFR2 amplification and in patient-derived gastric cancer xenografts, and the results were compared with short hairpin RNA knockdown of FGFR2 simultaneously. AZD4547 was found to inhibit phosphorylation of FGFR2 and downstream signaling molecules, including MAPK pathway in a dose-dependent manner,[10] and induced apoptosis in gastric cancer cell lines (KATO III and SNU-16) at inhibitory concentration (IC)50 values of 3 and 5 nmol/L, respectively. In contrast in the cell lines without FGFR2 amplification, there was insensitivity to AZD4547. Decrease in tumor growth in FGFR2-amplified xenograft models (SNU-16) was concordant with the tumor inhibition noted in vitro and in vivo using short hairpin RNA knockdown of FGFR2.[11] It was noted that treatment with AZF4547 over a 25-day period with daily doses of 12.5 mg/kg resulted in significant tumor regression in the xenograft models. Therefore, FGFR2 amplification seemed to be a valid predictive biomarker for AZD4547 in gastric cancer preclinical models.

With encouraging results from preclinical studies, a randomized phase 2 study was conducted comparing AZD4547 with weekly paclitaxel as a second-line or subsequent-line study.[12] Patients were preassigned to three groups based on FISH analysis of archival samples: (1) polysomy (FISH 4/5, ratio <2.0 and ≥4 copies in ≥10% cells), (2) low amplification (FISH6, ratio >2.0), and (3) high amplification (FISH6, ratio ≥5.0). Patients received either AZD4547, 80 mg orally twice daily for 2 weeks on and 1 week off in a 3-week cycle, or paclitaxel, 80 mg/m^2 intravenously weekly for 3 weeks of a 4-week cycle. The primary end point was progression free survival (PFS). In this study although AZD4547 was safe and well tolerated, there was no statistically significant difference in PFS between patients treated with AZD4547 or paclitaxel in either patients with FGFR2 polysomy or amplification. Close to 50% of recruited patients had polysomy rather than amplification; the latter was arguably the predictive biomarker identified in preclinical studies. Nevertheless there were no responders seen with the FGFR2 FISH6 group. In addition within this amplified group, there was still no PFS advantage seen with the AZD4547 compared with paclitaxel. Of note, the biomarker analysis showed that there was marked intratumoral heterogeneity of FGFR2 amplification and a low concordance with FGFR2 expression.

In a separate study AZD4547 was evaluated in a multicohort study, in patients with FGFR2 amplified gastric, esophageal, gastroesophageal junction (GOJ), adenocarcinoma, and FGFR1/2 amplified breast (HER2 negative) and squamous non–small cell lung cancers who had progressed through first-line and beyond of therapy.[8] This study was primarily designed for translational research to better understand the FGFR pathway, refine predictive biomarkers, and assess for resistance mechanisms. Patients were treated with either an intermittent schedule of 80 mg of AZD4547 twice daily, 2 weeks on and 1 week off in a 3-week cycle, or 80 mg of AZD4547 continuously, using Simon stage 2 design. FGFR1/2 amplification was tested centrally by FISH assay. Fluorodeoxyglucose (FDG) PET computed tomography at baseline, Day 14, and Week 8 of treatment; biopsy at baseline and biopsy on Day 14 to coincide with the FDG PET; and an optional biopsy on progression were performed. Phosphoimmunohistochemistry, FGFR copy number variation in tumor and plasma (circulating tumor DNA [ctDNA], using droplet digital polymerase chain reaction), and whole exome sequencing were performed as potential biomarkers assessments. Of the 285 patients screened, 132 patients with GOJ cancers were enrolled, of whom 9% were found to have FGFR2 amplification. Three of the nine patients responded with a concordant metabolic response noted on FDG PET, and the responses were durable (>29 weeks). AZD4547 was tolerated well with common adverse events (AEs) being fatigue (71%), mucositis (41%), nausea (35%), and nail changes (24%). Biopsies obtained at time of progression in nonresponders revealed acquired KRAS amplification. Interestingly, all patients who had a partial response had FGFR2 FISH ratio greater than 8 and elevated copy number as measured by ctDNA, whereas nonresponders did not have FGFR2 overamplification, suggesting that the level of amplification is crucial for response to therapy.

Reverse translation and further work at the bench on patient samples revealed that high-level, homogenous FGFR2 amplification (99% of tumor cells), as demonstrated by in situ heterogeneity mapping of FISH, was noted in the responders confirming that high-level clonal *FGFR2* amplification is a potential predictive biomarker of response to AZD4547. In a panel of 74 gastric cancer cell lines and tumors, a bimodal distribution of FGFR2 copy number was observed, with a distinct high-level FGFR2 amplified group, and in this group FGFR autophosphorylation was increased, in keeping with the high level of copy number, suggesting FGFR hyperactivation. FGFR2 copy number variation in plasma predicted response to AZD4547.[8]

In vitro experiments revealed that high-level amplification leads to distinct oncogene addiction and is characterized by FGFR2-mediated activation of other tyrosine receptor kinases, in particular FGFR-dependent control of the PI3K-mTOR pathway, through a noncanonical mechanism.[8] Of note, FGFR2 lacks a consensus-binding site for the PI3K regulatory subunit (p85), and FGFR2 overexpression activates PI3K signaling through other tyrosine kinases including through ERBB3 and IGF1R (insulin-like growth factor receptor-1); ERBB3 behaves as a scaffolding protein for the p85 subunit, whereas FGFR2 promotes RAS signaling and IGFR1 promotes binding of p85 via IRS1 (insulin receptor substrate-1) (**Fig. 1**). High-level FGFR2 amplification occurred in 5% (7 of 135, arbitrarily defined as FISH ratio >5) of gastric cancers in this study, and ctDNA can be used to screen patients with high-level FGFR2 amplification and is currently being used to enroll patients in this on-going study, making this the first study to use liquid biopsy for screening patients with gastric cancer. The study

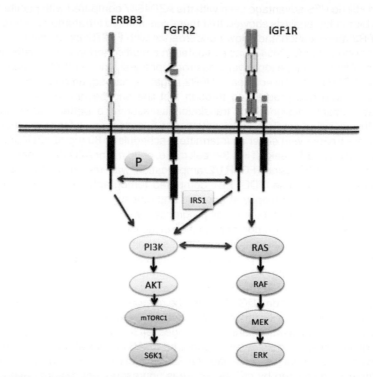

Fig. 1. FGFR2 amplification. High-level FGFR2 amplification causes an oncogene addiction phenotype. FGFR2 signals through other receptor tyrosine kinases; it transphosphorylates ERBB3, which acts as a scaffold for PI3K activating the PI3K pathway, and through insulin-like growth factor receptor (IGF1R) 1 activates PI3K pathway via RAS and insulin receptor substrate (IRS)-1.

has now been expanded as a basket study and is recruiting patients with any nonhematologic solid tumors with high-level FGFR2 amplification. **Table 1** provides details of ongoing studies with FGFR2 inhibitors.

Resistance to Fibroblast Growth Factor Receptor 2 Inhibitors

It is well established that there is redundancy in the tyrosine kinase family. Resistance to lapatanib, an oral HER2 inhibitor, is mediated through other tyrosine kinases, including MET, ERBB3, IGF1-R, and INSR. Similarly there is preclinical evidence to suggest that resistance to FGFR2 inhibitors is mediated through epithelial growth factor receptor (EGFR), ERBB3, and MET activation.[13,14] They form homodimers and heterodimers with each other and cross-phosphorylation of these tyrosine kinase receptors downstream signaling pathways, specifically the AKT-ERK pathway, and a common pathway that they all share. Epithelial growth factor (EGF) was noted to stimulate growth in the presence of FGFR inhibitor AZD4547, and this was associated with the reversal of the sub-G1 growth arrest that AZD4547 induces, and phosphorylation of downstream signaling pathway (AKT-ERK1/2) were noted on Western blotting. Synergistic activity was noted with decrease in tumor growth in vitro in gastric cell lines and in vivo in xenografts. Decrease in proliferative index (Ki67) and increase in apoptosis was noted, with EGFR positivity in the FGFR2 amplified tumors, and a role for combination therapy with FGFR2 inhibitor and EGFR inhibitor (cetuximab) has been postulated. FGFR2-amplified tumors were also noted to be copositive for ERBB3 (75% of tumors) and MET (25% of tumors) expression. This is particularly interesting because FGFR2 and HER2 amplification are mutually exclusive and it has been described that even when high-level amplifications co-occur, they do so in distinct areas of the tumor.[9]

Role of Fibroblast Growth Factor Receptor in Traztuzumab Resistance

Most patients with HER2-positive disease treated with traztuzumab develop resistance, usually within a year of therapy. In a study with HER2-amplified NCI-N87 orthotopic nude mouse model, traztuzumab resistance was induced and cell lines derived revealed HER2 down-regulation, with up-regulation of FGFR3 and induction of epithelial mesenchymal transition. Through clonal selection of FGFR3-amplified cells, signaling through PI3K/AKT/mTOR pathway confers survival and an aggressive epithelial mesenchymal transition phenotype. In preprogression and postprogression paired samples from patients treated with traztuzumab, overexpression of FGFR3 has been noted raising the possibility of the role of FGFR3 inhibitors, such as dovitinib, which inhibits phosphorylation of FGFR3, in patients with HER2-positive gastric adenocarcinoma who develop resistance to traztuzumab.[15]

CANCER STEM CELLS

Within the heterogeneous cancer populations are subpopulations of cells that have high tumorigenic potential, including the ability to metastasize, and are resistant to conventional chemotherapy and radiotherapy, by up-regulation of prosurvival and antiapoptotic signals, and increased DNA repair capacity and drug efflux receptors. Indeed, conventional treatments are thought to increase the degree of stemness in this group of cells. Gene silencing approaches have identified STAT3 as being critical in maintaining cancer stemness.

Signal Transducers and Activators of Transcription 3 Inhibitors

STAT proteins are a family of transcription factors that regulate cell proliferation, differentiation, angiogenesis, apoptosis, and immune and inflammatory responses.[16]

Table 1
Ongoing trials with novel agents

	Receptors Targeted	Phase of Study	Tumor Types Included	Line of Therapy	Study Design	Clinicaltrial.gov Number	Status
FGFR2 Inhibitors							
AZD4547	Highly selective FGFR1-3 inhibitor	Phase 2	Any solid tumor with FGFR2 amplification as tested by circulating DNA samples	Second line and beyond	AZD4547, 80 mg twice daily, 2 wk on, 1 wk off in a 21-d cycle	NCT01795768	Recruiting
Dovitinib	Dual VEGFR and FGFR inhibitor	Phase 1/2	Gastric adenocarcinoma	Second line and beyond	In combination with docetaxel In phase 1 portion of the study Docetaxel 45–75 mg/m^2, intravenous, every 3 wk Dovitinib 200–500 mg, oral, 5 d on/2 d off In phase 2 portion of the study recommended dose of docetaxel and dovitinib in phase 1 portion will be used	NCT01921673	Completed, report awaited
		Phase 2	Gastric adenocarcinoma with FGFR2 amplification	Second or third lines	500 mg once daily orally, 5 d on and 2 d off, weekly schedule	NCT01719549	Recruiting
Ponatinib	• FGFR1–FGFR4 • RET • PDGFR • FLT3 • VEGFR2 • bcr-abl • KIT	Phase 2	Solid tumors with genetic mutations of FGFR1, FGFR2, FGFR3, FGFR4, RET, KIT	Second line and beyond	Continuous once-daily administration, 28-d cycle	NCT02272998	Recruiting

FGFR and VEGF inhibitors

Lucitinib (E−3810)	Oral small molecule inhibitor of VEGFR1-3 and FGFR1	Phase 1/2a	All solid tumors	Second line and beyond	Continuous once-daily administration, 28-d cycle	NCT01283945	Ongoing but not recruiting participants
STAT3 inhibitors							
BBI608 (napabucasin)	Oral small molecule STAT3 inhibitor	Phase 3	Gastric and gastroesophageal junction adenocarcinoma	Second line and beyond 1	BBI608 with weekly paclitaxel vs weekly paclitaxel	NCT02178956	Recruiting
		Phase 1b	Advanced gastrointestinal tumors	First line and beyond	BBI608 administered orally, continuously in combination with standard treatments (FOLFOX or FOLFOX with bevacizumab or CAPOX or FOLFIRI or FOLFIRI with bevacizumab or with regorafenib or single agent irinotecan	NCT02024607	Recruiting
		Phase 1/2	Any advanced solid tumor		BBI608 in combination with immune checkpoint inhibitors (ipilimumab, nivolumab, and pembrolizumab)	NCT02467361	Recruiting

(continued on next page)

Table 1
(continued)

	Receptors Targeted	Phase of Study	Tumor Types Included	Line of Therapy	Study Design	Clinicaltrial.gov Number	Status
CLDN18.2 inhibitors							
IMAB362	CLDN18.2 inhibitor	Phase 2	Patients with CLDN18.2-positive gastric, esophageal or gastroesophageal junction adenocarcinomas	First line	IMAB362 in combination with the EOX regimen	NCT01630083	Completed recruitment
Matrix metalloproteinase-9 inhibitors							
GS-5745	MMP-9 antibody	Phase 3	Patients with advanced gastric or gastroesophageal junction adenocarcinomas	First line	GS-5745 800 mg intravenously every 2 wk with mFOLFOX6	NCT02545504	Recruiting

Data from ClinicalTrials.gov. US National Institutes of Health. Available at: https://clinicaltrials.gov/. Accessed on August 31, 2016.

STAT3 hyperactivation has been noted in 30% to 70% gastric cancers and is correlated to differentiation, stage of disease, lymph node metastases, and poor prognosis.[17] It is also thought to be the key for cancer cells to maintain their stemness.[18,19] Trials focusing on targeting the upstream signaling pathways of STAT3 including blocking Janus activated kinase have not been entirely successful.

Constitutive activation of STAT3 was noted in gastric cancer cell lines and inhibition of STAT3 induced apoptosis, decreased cell proliferation, and affected G-G2 cell cycle transition by affecting cyclin D1. STAT3 activation was found to be crucial in initiation and development of distal gastric adenocarcinoma in mouse models. Other preclinical studies have corroborated the role of STAT3 in tumorigenesis, progression by affecting cyclin D1 and c-myc, survival and by affecting MMP-13, the extracellular matrix degradation increasing the metastatic potential.[20]

Cancer stem cells are thought to be mediate resistance to chemotherapy and targeted agents and responsible for metastases. Napabucasin (BBI608), a first-in-class, small-molecule-inhibitor of STAT3, showed inhibition of spheroid formation and down-regulation of genes associated with stemness including c-myc and β-catenin (**Fig. 2**).[19] Nanog, Axl, Sox-2, Klf4, surviving, and Bmi protein levels showed a dose– dependent decrease. Normal stem cells were not affected as demonstrated by the lack of inhibition of colony formation by hematopoietic stem cells (CD34$^+$) even at high concentrations. Stemness-high stem cells responded better to BBI608 than other cells in a heterogeneous population of cancer cells. With regard to nonstem cancer cells acquiring stemness, BBI608 prevented relapse and metastases in in vivo pancreatic models treated with conventional chemotherapy. Napabucasin combined with paclitaxel was observed to have synergistic antitumor effect.

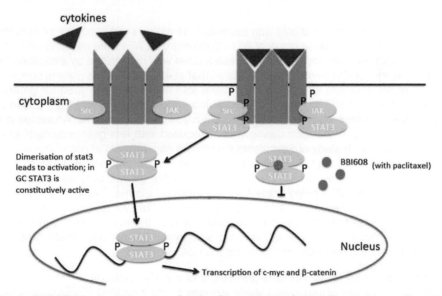

Fig. 2. STAT3 inhibitors. STAT3 are a family of transcription factors that regulate cell proliferation, differentiation, angiogenesis, apoptosis, immune and inflammatory responses, and stemness. Constitutive activation of STAT3 is noted in 30% to 70% of patients with GC. In GC cell lines inhibition of STAT3 by small molecule inhibitor BBI608, with paclitaxel, induced apoptosis, decreased cell proliferation, and affected G-G2 cell cycle transition by affecting cyclin D1. Decreased transcription of genes associated with stemness, including c-myc and β-catenin, was noted.

In HER2-positive gastric cancer cell line NCI-N87R resistance to traztuzumab was induced by prolonged exposure to traztuzumab. In the subclones an increase in phosphorylation of STAT3 compared with the parental cell line was noted. Treatment with Jak2/STAT3 inhibitors reversed the resistance but inhibitors of more upstream proteins (PI3K and MAPK inhibitors) had no effect,[21] perhaps because STAT3 are constitutively active. Three compounds (OPB-31121, OPB-51602, and napabucasin) have been tested to date. Ongoing studies are summarized in **Table 1**.

OPB-31121

In a phase 1 study[22] of 39 patients with advanced treatment-refractory solid tumors, OPB-31121 at dose levels between 50 and 350 mg was administered twice daily for 21 days in a 28-day cycle and 300 mg was found to be the maximum tolerated dose (MTD). No objective responses were observed and patients experienced rapid disease progression; toxicities were all grade 1 to 2, with nausea, vomiting, and diarrhea being common side effects.

OPB-51602

OPB-51602 is an orally active inhibitor of phosphorylation of STAT3. In a single arm phase 1 study of 51 Asian patients with refractory advanced malignancies,[23] patients were treated in three cohorts. Patients in cohort A had OPB- 51602 administered on an intermittent schedule at dose levels 2, 4, and 5 mg. The MTD was 5 mg. Cohort B was a dose expansion of 4 mg. Patients in cohort C received 4 mg of the drug continuously in 28-day cycles. Overall the compound was found to be safe and tolerable with common AEs being nausea, vomiting, anorexia, reversible peripheral neuropathy, and fatigue; in cohort C, 16% developed grade 3/4 AEs.

Napabucasin (BBI608)

In a phase 1 study of 41 patients with treatment-refractory solid tumors,[24] 14 cohorts were dosed through a dose range of 20 to 2000 mg/day. AEs were mild and an MTD was not reached. The recommended phase 2 dose was determined by evaluation of pharmacokinetics (PK) levels, which revealed that at 400 mg/day, the plasma concentration of napabucasin was sustained several fold higher than the IC50 for greater than 8 hours, and 500 mg/day was carried forward as the recommended phase 2 dose. Objective response rate (ORR) was observed in 65% of patients. An expansion study[25] found that twice-daily dosing was associated with less gastrointestinal side effects. A phase 1b study of 24 patients combining napabucasin at escalating doses of 200, 400, and 500 mg twice daily with paclitaxel at 80 mg/m^2 administered weekly for 3 weeks of a 4-week cycle[26] revealed that the 500-mg twice daily was well tolerated with common AEs being grade 1/2, and included diarrhea, abdominal cramps, nausea, and vomiting. Grade 3 AEs included diarrhea, dehydration, and weakness. A total of 67% of patients had disease control and of the five patients with gastric or GOJ tumors, two had partial response and three patients had stable disease, two of whom had stable disease for more than 24 weeks.

Combination study of napabucasin (BBI-608) and weekly paclitaxel

Based on the results of the phase 1 study, a phase 2 extension study[26] was conducted in 46 patients with pretreated (one or more lines of treatment) metastatic gastric and GOJ adenocarcinoma. Patients were treated with BBI-608 at 480 mg or 500 mg, orally, twice daily with paclitaxel 80 mg/m^2 intravenously weekly for 3 of a 4-week cycle. The study population included patients with HER2 amplified disease who had received traztuzumab. In 78% of patients, this combination was their third-line therapy. In 20 patients who had not received a taxane in the metastatic setting, the

ORR was 31% with a median PFS of 20.6 weeks and median OS of 39.3 weeks; in 26 patients who had previously received taxane (median three lines of prior therapy), the ORR was 11% with a median PFS of 12.6 weeks and median OS of 33.1 weeks. In six patients who received only one prior, nontaxane therapy, the ORR was 50%. The tolerability of the combination was good and AEs were grade 1/2 diarrhea, abdominal cramps, nausea, and vomiting. Grade 3 AEs included vomiting in 9% of patients and diarrhea and fatigue in 7% of patients.

Based on these findings, the phase-3 BRIGHTER study (NCT02178956) is evaluating this combination in patients with gastric and GOJ adenocarcinomas following progression through first-line platinum-based therapy and the results of this multicenter, randomized, placebo-controlled trail are eagerly awaited. The study aims to recruit 680 patients in a 1:1 randomization with patients randomized to either napabucasin administered twice daily with weekly paclitaxel (80 mg/m^2 every week for 3 of a 4-week cycle) or placebo with weekly paclitaxel. The primary end point is OS with secondary objectives of PFS, ORR, disease control rate, PK, and quality of life. β-catenin levels by immunohistochemistry are being measured to explore correlation between drug exposure and response.[27]

CLDN18.2 INHIBITORS

The claudin family, composed of at least 24 transmembrane proteins, is a major component of tight junctions. They are ubiquitous, form homodimers and heterodimers and create epithelial sheets, and are present in normal gastric mucosa; claudins 1, 3, 4, and 5 are expressed in 70% to 90% of gastric cancers. Expression of claudin 3 is associated with better prognosis[28] and loss of claudin expression, in particular, claudin 18 isoform 2, is more common in diffuse type of gastric cancers much more than intestinal type, and is associated with poor prognosis.[29] From the Cancer Genome Atlas, RNA sequencing data revealed interchromosomal translocation between CLDN18.2 and ARHGAP26, and CLDN18.2-ARHGAP26 fusions leading to dysregulated RHO signaling, which is crucial for cell motility and cellular cohesion.[14] Disruption of wild-type CLDN18.2 also impacts on cellular adhesion, and it is thought that these genetic changes lead to the invasive phenotype of diffuse gastric cancers.

IMB362 is an investigational medicinal product targeting claudin 18 isoform 2 (CLDN18.2). Anti-CLDN18.2 antibodies through antibody-dependent cellular cytotoxicity and complement-dependent cytotoxicity in combination with chemotherapy are thought to enhance T-cell infiltration and induce proinflammatory cytokines[16,30] (Fig. 3).

The FAST study is a multicenter, randomized, first-line, phase 2 study of chemotherapy (EOX-epirubicin, 50 mg/m^2 every 3 week; oxaliplatin, 130 mg/m^2 every 3 weeks; and capecitabine, 1250 mg/m^2 days 1–21 of each cycle) with or without IMB362 antibody (800 mg/m2 loading and 600 mg/m^2 every 3 weeks) in patients with locally advanced or metastatic CLDN18.2$^+$ (either 2$^+$ or 3$^+$ in >40% of tumor cells) gastric or GOJ adenocarcinoma.[31] A total of 730 patients were enrolled of whom CLDN18.2 expression was evaluable in 686 patients, and about 45% were deemed CLDN18.2 positive. The initial randomization was 1:1, and a further exploratory cohort was added with patients receiving 1000 mg/m^2 of the anti-CLDN18.2 antibody. The primary end point was PFS comparing IMAB362 (800/600 mg/m^2) with EOX versus EOX alone. Of the 252 patients randomized, 246 patients received treatment, 84 received chemotherapy alone, 77 patients EOX + IMAB362 at a dose of 800/600 mg/m^2, and 85 EOX + IMAB362 at a dose of 1000 mg/m^2. IMAB362 was found to be tolerable. PFS was 4.8 months in the chemotherapy group and

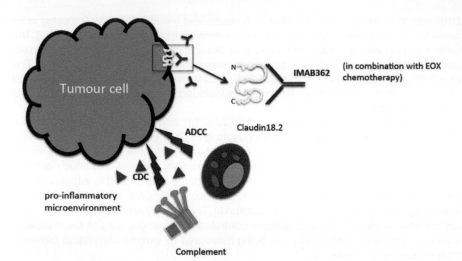

Fig. 3. Claudin 18.2 inhibitors. The claudin family is a major component of tight junctions, they create epithelial sheets, are present in normal gastric mucosa, and loss of claudin 18 isoform 2 is common in diffuse type of gastric cancers. Anti-CLDN18.2 antibodies, IMAB362, through antibody-dependent cellular cytotoxicity (ADCC) and complement-dependent cytotoxicity (CDC) in combination with chemotherapy are thought to enhance T-cell infiltration and induce proinflammatory cytokines.

7.9 months (hazard ratio [HR], 0.47; 95% confidence interval [CI], 0.31–0.70; P = .0001) in patients treated with the antibody-chemotherapy combination. In patients in arm 3, PFS was 7.1 months with an HR of 0.51 (P = .001). OS was 13.2 months in IMAB362 800/600 mg/m2 compared with 8.4 months in the chemotherapy arm (HR, 0.51; P = .0001). Subset analysis of patients whose tumors had high expression of CLDN18.2 ($\geq$70% of tumor cells) revealed that the median PFS was 7.2 months versus 5.6 (HR, 0.36; $P<$.0005) and median OS was 16.7 months versus 9 months (HR, 0.45; $P<$.0005) in IMAB 362 versus chemotherapy arm, respectively. Common AEs with the IMAB 362 + EOX combination included vomiting and uncomplicated neutropenia.

MATRIX METALLOPROTEINASE INHIBITORS

MMPs are a family of zinc-dependent, extracellular matrix and basement membrane endopeptidases. At least 28 MMPs have been identified to date, and normally they play a crucial role in tissue remodeling. The genes encoding MMPs only become transcriptionally active when tissue modeling is required, and the protein is secreted in a pro-MMP form. The peptide domain of the pro-MMPs is cleaved by proteases allowing for hydrolysis of the zinc moiety, and this triggers autocatalytic cleavage of the pro-peptide domain activating the MMP. Tissue inhibitors called TIMPs heavily regulate activity of MMPs. MMP-2, -7, -9, and -14 are overexpressed in patients with gastric cancer and MMP-9 have been implicated in cancer metastases and tumor angiogenesis,[32] and by paracrine signaling to stromal cells affects the tumor microenvironment[33] (Fig. 4). MMP inhibitors have shown inhibition of tumor growth in human gastric cancer in xenograft models. Historically, several nonspecific MMP inhibitors including marimastat have been tested with small clinical benefit and side effect profile limiting their use. We now have specific MMP-9 inhibitors that have been developed and are in clinical trials in patients with GC.

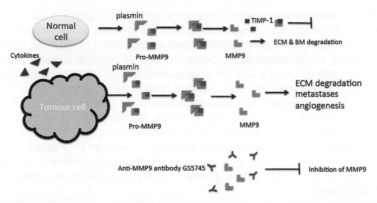

Fig. 4. MMP-9 inhibitors are a family of zinc-dependent, extracellular matrix (ECM) and basement membrane (BM) endopeptidases and play a crucial role in tissue remodeling. The genes encoding MMPs only become transcriptionally active when tissue modeling is required; the protein is secreted in a pro-MMP form. The peptide domain of the pro-MMPs is cleaved by proteases (plasmin) activating the MMP. Tissue inhibitors called TIMPs heavily regulate activity of MMPs. In the tumor microenvironment, there is unregulated MMP production leading to ECM degradation, metastases, and angiogenesis. Specific anti-MMP-9 antibody GS5745 is currently in clinical trials.

Marimastat

Marimastat is a broad-spectrum, reversible inhibitor of MMPs (MMP-1, -2, -3, -7, -9, and -12). In a pilot study[34] of marimastat in patients with advanced gastric cancer, patients received treatment for a period of 28 days, safety and tolerability were evaluated, and the endoscopic assessment of their gastric tumor was performed. Thirty-five patients were recruited, of whom 29 had stage 4 disease. They were treated at a starting dose of 50 mg twice daily, which was reduced to 25 mg once daily (29 of the 35 patients received this dose). The drug was tolerated well; musculoskeletal pain and stiffness associated with inflammation was the most common AE, and was reversible on drug interruption. Following on from the pilot study, a randomized double-blind, placebo-controlled study[35] of marimastat was performed to assess whether MMP inhibitor showed benefit as maintenance therapy in patients with nonresectable gastric and gastroesophageal adenocarcinoma, who had received first line 5-FU. A total of 369 patients were enrolled to receive oral marimastat (10 mg twice daily) or a placebo, and were treated as long as they tolerated treatment. Primary end point was OS with time to disease progression and quality of life being secondary end points. A modest difference in survival in favor of marimastat was noted in the intention-to-treat population (P = .07; HR, 1.23; 95% CI, 0.98–1.55). Follow-up over a period of 2 years revealed that the survival benefit was maintained, with a median OS of 160 days for the trial arm and 138 days with the placebo, with a similar increase in PFS noted. Musculoskeletal pain and inflammation were common side effects with the drug.

Specific Matrix Metalloproteinase 9 Inhibitors

In a phase 1 study of GS-5745, a humanized monoclonal antibody of MMP-9, in 88 patients with advanced solid tumors, the antibody was used alone in the dose-escalation phase up to 1800 mg intravenously every 2 weeks, and in the dose-expansion phase in patients with esophagogastric adenocarcinoma at a dose of 800 mg intravenously every 2 weeks in combination with mFOLFOX6 (modified leucovorin, 5-FU, and oxaliplatin) regimen.[36,37] Thirty-nine patients with gastric (17 patients) and GOJ (23 patients) adenocarcinomas were enrolled, 37 patients had metastatic disease, and three patients had locally advanced disease. In the treatment-naive group (29 patients), 64% of patients had objective response to treatment, 55% of patients achieving partial response or better and three patients achieving complete response (two with no target lesions and one patient with target lesion at baseline). Uncomplicated myelosuppression, nausea, and fatigue were common AEs. The most common treatment-emergent AEs were abdominal pain, gastrointestinal hemorrhage, hyponatremia, nausea, pyrexia, and septic shock. Median PFS was 12 months (90% CI, 5.5–18.0) in the treatment-naive group, and 4.8 months (90% CI, 1.7–13.9) in previously treated groups.[37] Levels of C1M, a product of cleavage of collagen-1 by MMP, correlated with treatment responses, and was identified as a potential biomarker of response. Based on these data, a phase 3 study is currently recruiting patients (**Table 1** for details).

SUMMARY

The progress being made with new agents in treatment of advanced gastric cancer is exciting for patients and the clinical community. Combination treatment strategies with conventional chemotherapies, and targeted agents including immune checkpoint inhibitors are also being explored. In developing novel therapeutics in treatment of patients with GC/GOC, it is clear that parallel research efforts to refine target population and biomarkers are crucial. Reverse translation with clinically relevant biospecimens studied back at the bench is important to understand the biology and the mechanism of action, but also to evaluate the mechanisms of resistance. It is hoped that the molecular characterization of not just the tumor, but also its interaction with the tumor microenvironment leading to coevolution of tumor-stromal components will have an impact on future treatments.

ACKNOWLEDGMENTS

The authors thank National Health Service for funding to the National Institute for Health Research Biomedical Research Centre at the Royal Marsden NHS Foundation Trust and the Institute of Cancer Research.

REFERENCES

1. Ferlay J, Soerjomataram I, Dikshit R, et al. Cancer incidence and mortality worldwide: sources, methods and major patterns in GLOBOCAN 2012. Int J Cancer 2015;136(5):E359–86.
2. Hanahan D, Weinberg RA. Hallmarks of cancer: the next generation. Cell 2011; 144(5):646–74.
3. Jang JH, Shin KH, Park JG. Mutations in fibroblast growth factor receptor 2 and fibroblast growth factor receptor 3 genes associated with human gastric and colorectal cancers. Cancer Res 2001;61(9):3541–3.
4. Jemal A, Bray F, Center MM, et al. Global cancer statistics. CA Cancer J Clin 2011;61(2):69–90.
5. Turner N, Grose R. Fibroblast growth factor signalling: from development to cancer. Nat Rev Cancer 2010;10(2):116–29.
6. Hattori Y, Itoh H, Uchino S, et al. Immunohistochemical detection of K-sam protein in stomach cancer. Clin Cancer Res 1996;2(8):1373–81.
7. Matsumoto K, Arao T, Hamaguchi T, et al. FGFR2 gene amplification and clinicopathological features in gastric cancer. Br J Cancer 2012;106(4):727–32.

8. Pearson A, Smyth E, Babina IS, et al. High-level clonal FGFR amplification and response to FGFR inhibition in a translational clinical trial. Cancer Discov 2016; 6(8):838–51.

9. Su X, Zhan P, Gavine PR, et al. FGFR2 amplification has prognostic significance in gastric cancer: results from a large international multicentre study. Br J Cancer 2014;110(4):967–75.

10. Gavine PR, Mooney L, Kilgour E, et al. AZD4547: an orally bioavailable, potent, and selective inhibitor of the fibroblast growth factor receptor tyrosine kinase family. Cancer Res 2012;72(8):2045–56.

11. Xie L, Su X, Zhang L, et al. FGFR2 gene amplification in gastric cancer predicts sensitivity to the selective FGFR inhibitor AZD4547. Clin Cancer Res 2013;19(9): 2572–83.

12. Bang Y-J, Van Cutsem E, Mansoor W, et al. A randomized, open-label phase II study of AZD4547 (AZD) versus paclitaxel (P) in previously treated patients with advanced gastric cancer (AGC) with fibroblast growth factor receptor 2 (FGFR2) polysomy or gene amplification (amp): SHINE study. ASCO Meeting Abstracts 2015;33(15_Suppl):4014.

13. Chang J, Wang S, Zhang Z, et al. Multiple receptor tyrosine kinase activation attenuates therapeutic efficacy of the fibroblast growth factor receptor 2 inhibitor AZD4547 in FGFR2 amplified gastric cancer. Oncotarget 2015;6(4):2009–22.

14. Cancer Genome Atlas Research Network. Comprehensive molecular characterization of gastric adenocarcinoma. Nature 2014;513(7517):202–9.

15. Piro G, Carbone C, Cataldo I, et al. An FGFR3 autocrine loop sustains acquired resistance to trastuzumab in gastric cancer patients. Clin Cancer Res 2016; 22(24):6164–75.

16. Cafferkey C, Chau I. Novel STAT 3 inhibitors for treating gastric cancer. Expert Opin Investig Drugs 2016;25(9):1023–31.

17. Lee J, Kang WK, Park JO, et al. Expression of activated signal transducer and activator of transcription 3 predicts poor clinical outcome in gastric adenocarcinoma. APMIS 2009;117(8):598–606.

18. Deng JY, Sun D, Liu XY, et al. STAT-3 correlates with lymph node metastasis and cell survival in gastric cancer. World J Gastroenterol 2010;16(42):5380–7.

19. Li Y, Rogoff HA, Keates S, et al. Suppression of cancer relapse and metastasis by inhibiting cancer stemness. Proc Natl Acad Sci U S A 2015;112(6):1839–44.

20. Ernst M, Najdovska M, Grail D, et al. STAT3 and STAT1 mediate IL-11-dependent and inflammation-associated gastric tumorigenesis in gp130 receptor mutant mice. J Clin Invest 2008;118(5):1727–38.

21. Yang Z, Guo L, Liu D, et al. Acquisition of resistance to trastuzumab in gastric cancer cells is associated with activation of IL-6/STAT3/Jagged-1/Notch positive feedback loop. Oncotarget 2015;6(7):5072–87.

22. Bendell JC, Hong DS, Burris HA 3rd, et al. Phase 1, open-label, dose-escalation, and pharmacokinetic study of STAT3 inhibitor OPB-31121 in subjects with advanced solid tumors. Cancer Chemother Pharmacol 2014;74(1):125–30.

23. Wong AL, Soo RA, Tan DS, et al. Phase I and biomarker study of OPB-51602, a novel signal transducer and activator of transcription (STAT) 3 inhibitor, in patients with refractory solid malignancies. Ann Oncol 2015;26(5):998–1005.

24. Langleben A, Supko JG, Hotte SJ, et al. A dose-escalation phase I study of a first-in-class cancer stemness inhibitor in patients with advanced malignancies. ASCO Meeting Abstracts 2013;31(15_Suppl):2542.

25. Jonker DJ, Stephenson J, Edenfield WJ, et al. A phase I extension study of BBI608, a first-in-class cancer stem cell (CSC) inhibitor, in patients with advanced solid tumors. ASCO Meeting Abstracts 2014;32(15_Suppl):2546.

26. Hitron M, Stephenson J, Chi KN, et al. A phase 1b study of the cancer stem cell inhibitor BBI608 administered with paclitaxel in patients with advanced malignancies. ASCO Meeting Abstracts 2014;32(15_Suppl):2530.

27. Shah MA, Muro K, Shitara K, et al. The BRIGHTER trial: a phase III randomized double-blind study of BBI608 + weekly paclitaxel versus placebo (PBO) + weekly paclitaxel in patients (pts) with pretreated advanced gastric and gastroesophageal junction (GEJ) adenocarcinoma. ASCO Meeting Abstracts 2015; 33(15_Suppl):TPS4139.

28. Soini Y, Tommola S, Helin H, et al. Claudins 1, 3, 4 and 5 in gastric carcinoma, loss of claudin expression associates with the diffuse subtype. Virchows Arch 2006;448(1):52–8.

29. Jun KH, Kim JH, Jung JH, et al. Expression of claudin-7 and loss of claudin-18 correlate with poor prognosis in gastric cancer. Int J Surg 2014;12(2):156–62.

30. Rogers LM, Veeramani S, Weiner GJ. Complement in monoclonal antibody therapy of cancer. Immunol Res 2014;59(1–3):203–10.

31. Al-Batran S-E, Schuler MH, Zvirbule Z, et al. FAST: an international, multicenter, randomized, phase II trial of epirubicin, oxaliplatin, and capecitabine (EOX) with or without IMAB362, a first-in-class anti-CLDN18.2 antibody, as first-line therapy in patients with advanced CLDN18.2+ gastric and gastroesophageal junction (GEJ) adenocarcinoma. ASCO Meeting Abstracts 2016;34(15_Suppl): LBA4001.

32. Bergers G, Brekken R, McMahon G, et al. Matrix metalloproteinase-9 triggers the angiogenic switch during carcinogenesis. Nat Cell Biol 2000;2(10):737–44.

33. Marshall DC, Lyman SK, McCauley S, et al. Selective allosteric inhibition of MMP9 is efficacious in preclinical models of ulcerative colitis and colorectal cancer. PLoS One 2015;10(5):e0127063.

34. Tierney GM, Griffin NR, Stuart RC, et al. A pilot study of the safety and effects of the matrix metalloproteinase inhibitor marimastat in gastric cancer. Eur J Cancer 1999;35(4):563–8.

35. Bramhall SR, Hallissey MT, Whiting J, et al. Marimastat as maintenance therapy for patients with advanced gastric cancer: a randomised trial. Br J Cancer 2002;86(12):1864–70.

36. Bendell JC, Starodub A, Shah MA, et al. Phase I study of GS-5745 alone and in combination with chemotherapy in patients with advanced solid tumors. ASCO Meeting Abstracts 2015;33(15_Suppl):4030.

37. Shah MA, Starodub A, Wainberg ZA, et al. Results of a phase I study of GS-5745 in combination with mFOLFOX in patients with advanced unresectable gastric/ GE junction tumors. ASCO Meeting Abstracts 2016;34(15_Suppl):4033.

Future Directions in Improving Outcomes for Patients with Gastric and Esophageal Cancer

Manish A. Shah, MD

KEYWORDS

- Molecular profiling • Epidemiology • *Helicobacter pylori* • Targeted therapy
- Locally advanced disease

KEY POINTS

- Over the past 10 years, we have witnessed dramatic changes in both our understanding of gastric and esophageal cancer, in particular that disease subtypes exist and now applying this knowledge to clinical utility, as well as its management, in particular with the use of adjuvant therapy for locally advanced disease and multiple lines of treatment of patients with metastatic disease.
- We are no longer limited to cytotoxic systemic therapy, as we have 2 new biological agents approved to treat advanced disease, with several more promising prospects under development.
- In this article, the author looks to the future, attempting to answer the question of which advancements will play the biggest role in improving patient outcomes in this still-devastating disease.

INTRODUCTION

As this issue of *Hematology/Oncology Clinics of North America* has outlined, there have been many advances in understanding the molecular underpinnings of gastric and esophageal cancer and how these cancers are now managed. However, despite the many advances in the management of gastric and esophageal cancers discussed herein, the reality remains that most patients diagnosed with gastric or esophageal cancer will ultimately die of their disease, most living for less than 1 year once their disease has metastasized. In countries apart from Japan and Korea, for example, those without an active gastric cancer screening program, most patients with gastric and esophageal cancer will be diagnosed with locally advanced or metastatic disease.[1]

Weill Cornell Medicine/New York-Presbyterian Hospital, Division of Hematology and Medical Oncology, 1305 York Avenue, New York, NY 10021, USA
E-mail address: mas9313@med.cornell.edu

Hematol Oncol Clin N Am 31 (2017) 545–552
http://dx.doi.org/10.1016/j.hoc.2017.01.010
0889-8588/17/© 2017 Elsevier Inc. All rights reserved.
hemonc.theclinics.com

Patients with locally advanced disease are more likely to have micrometastatic disease that results in higher rates of recurrence, usually within 2 years, following resection of the primary disease. These sobering data likely explain some of the differences in the epidemiology and natural course between cancers identified on screening and sporadic gastric cancers. Indeed, in the United States, the fatality/case ratio for gastroesophageal cancers is 0.66,[2] suggesting that approximately two-thirds of newly diagnosed patients will have metastatic disease at some point during the course of their illness and will require systemic therapy.

Many drugs are considered active in the treatment of gastric and esophageal cancer, including platinum (cisplatin and oxaliplatin), fluoropyrimidines, irinotecan, taxanes, and targeted therapies (ie, trastuzumab and ramucirumab).[3] It is compelling that we have approval of 2 new targeted antibody approaches to the disease in the past several years. However, despite the many treatment options available, median survival for advanced gastric cancer remains 8 to 10 months for most patients.[4,5] There are several areas where the author thinks that advances can possibly alter these harsh realities.

DISEASE PREVENTION

Gastric cancer is responsible for approximately 952,000 new diagnoses (6.8% of new cancer cases worldwide) and 723,000 deaths annually (8.8% of total).[6] In the United States in 2009, an estimated 21,130 new cases (14th most common) of gastric cancer were diagnosed with 10,620 deaths (13th most common). In Europe, gastric cancer ranks fifth with an estimated 159,900 new cases per year in 2006 and 118,200 deaths (fourth most common cause of cancer-related death).[7] Nearly two-thirds of all cases globally occur in developing countries in Eastern Europe, South America, and Asia, with 42% of all new cases developed in China alone.[8]

Gastric cancer is a heterogeneous disease with several established risk factors (summarized by Shah[5]). Gastric cancer subtypes (proximal nondiffuse, diffuse, and distal nondiffuse)[5] defined by these risk factors have been molecularly classified as unique entities.[9] The most relevant hereditable causes of gastric cancer include constitutional mutations in CDH1 (causing hereditary diffuse gastric cancer[10]) and DNA repair enzyme deficiency in Lynch syndrome.[11] Individuals carrying a CDH1 mutation have an 80% lifetime risk of developing gastric cancer and are, therefore, recommended to undergo a risk-reducing prophylactic gastrectomy.[12] However, environmental or modifiable factors are also major contributors to the development of this disease.[5,13] For example, in a study of cancer risk in monozygotic and dizygotic twins, the estimated proportion of nonshared environmental factors contributing to gastric cancer risk is 62%, whereas the contribution from heritable risk is estimated at only 28%.[14]

The most significant environmental risk factor is infection with Helicobacter pylori, a gram-negative bacillus identified in 1983 as the pathogen responsible for gastric ulcers and peptic ulcer disease. H pylori is the most common chronic bacterial pathogen in humans,[15] with a high prevalence in both developing and industrialized countries. In 1994, the World Health Organization and the International Agency for Research on Cancer consensus group classified H pylori as a class I carcinogen.[16] Notably, however, less than 1% of infected patients develop gastric cancer during their lifetime.[17] The bacterium is present in the stomachs of at least half of the world's population and is usually acquired in childhood. When left untreated, the pathogen generally persists for the individuals' lifetime. Therefore, exposure to H pylori is chronic and long-standing. This long latency period between infection and the development of malignancy may provide an opportunity to impact on the development of the disease by possibly providing opportunity to intervene to prevent progressive accumulation of cell damage.[18] Understanding the mucosal microenvironmental changes that lead to carcinogenesis will be a key factor in identifying who may benefit from screening programs. In this regard, the microbiome of the stomach and its impact on mucosal immunity are areas that will come to the forefront as we think about improving are strategies for disease prevention.

MOLECULAR CLASSIFICATION OF DISEASE

Understanding disease subtypes to improve enrichment strategies for targeted therapy will be another transformative area in managing gastric and esophageal cancers. The Cancer Genome Atlas analysis has defined 4 major subtypes of gastric cancer.[19] Chromosomal instability and mismatch repair subtypes are two major classes of gastric cancer that may be related to *H pylori* infection. The other important subtypes of gastric cancer include genomically stable and Epstein-Barr virus (EBV) subtypes of gastric cancer. Each subtype is molecularly unique, with implications for drug development.

Gastric cancers with chromosomal instability are associated with *TP53* mutation with receptor tyrosine kinase (RTK)-RA + Sarcoma oncogene homologue (RAS) activation. This subtype of gastric cancer is most closely related to the intestinal subtype. The high rate (~70%) of *TP53* mutations is associated with a high level of somatic copy number variations identified in both focal gene regions as well as at the chromosomal level.[20] The RTK-RAS mutations may offer another opportunity to target. Specifically, it has been demonstrated in other tumor models that high-dose ascorbate may preferentially target RAS-driven tumors.[21]

The EBV type is reported to represent around 10% of gastric cancers and harbors a higher prevalence of DNA hypermethylation than the other subtypes, likely specifically related to EBV infection.[22] This subtype has a high prevalence (~80%) of mutations in *PIK3CA*, overexpression of programmed death ligand 1 (PD-L1) and PD-L2, EBV-CpG island methylator phenotype (CIMP) expression, and *CDKN2A* silencing, as well as altered cytokine signaling.[19]

Patients with microsatellite instable gastric cancer present at an older age; their tumors exhibit moderate genomic hypermutation, gastric CIMP, *MLH1* silencing, and varying mitotic pathways. This subtype, as a consequence of defective mismatch repair due to *MLH1* silencing secondary to promoter hypermethylation, has a significantly greater number of mutations per megabase than other types of gastric cancer.[19] This circumstance would predict increased efficacy with checkpoint inhibitor immunotherapy[23]; however, there is no consensus on the definition of microsatellite instability in gastric cancer at this time. A detailed discussion of immunotherapy in gastroesophageal cancers is provided in Drs Adrian G. Murphy and Ronan J. Kelly's article, "The Evolving Role of Checkpoint Inhibitors in the Management of Gastroesophageal Cancer," in this issue.

Finally, the genomically stable gastric cancer subtype is enriched for Lauren's diffuse histology, *CDH1* and *RHOA* mutations, cell adhesion, and Claudin-18 – Rho GTPase-activating protein 1 (*CLDN18*-ARHGAP) fusion. Germline mutations in *CDH1* are responsible for the genetic predisposition syndrome, hereditary diffuse gastric cancer (HDGC). The lifetime risk of developing HDGC for a *CDH1* mutation carrier has recently been estimated at 70% (95% confidence interval [CI], 59%–80%) for men and 56% (95% CI, 44%–69%) for women, and the risk of breast cancer for women was 42% (95% CI, 23%–68%)[24] similar to the risk of developing breast cancer in women who carry some BRCA mutations.[10,25] Because the risk is so high, prophylactic gastrectomy is recommended by the International Gastric Cancer Linkage Consortium after 20 years of age for people who are known *CDH1* mutation carriers.[26,27] Increased awareness of genetic predisposition syndromes will improve patient outcomes in this disease, though the impact is likely to be low, given that an estimated only 10% to 15% of gastric cancers are thought to be related to a constitutional gene mutation. Another identifiable, and potentially targetable, mutation in the genomically stable gastric cancer subtype is the *CLDN18-ARHGAP6* or *26* fusion.[28] This fusion further strengthens the implication of alterations in Rho signaling and the significance of cell adhesion in this subtype of gastric cancer because *CLDN18* is involved in intercellular tight junctions and ARHGAP26 is a GTPase-activating protein that activates Rho signaling by facilitating the conversion of Rho GTPases to the GDP state.[29] As reported in Drs Gayathri Anandappa and Ian Chau's article, "Emerging Novel Therapeutic Agents in the Treatment of Patients with Gastroesophageal and Gastric Adenocarcinoma," in this issue, *CLDN18.2* inhibition is a promising new target in treating gastric cancer.

The characterization of gastric cancer into specific disease subtypes is the beginning of the application of precision medicine to gastric and esophageal cancers. It is anticipated that, with improving our ability to subgroup gastric cancer in real time, and by using these data to direct treatment, we will make significant strides in improving patient outcomes.

IMPROVE OUTCOMES IN PATIENTS WITH LOCALLY ADVANCED DISEASE

It is recognized that therapies that effectively treat micrometastatic disease will have the greatest impact on patient outcomes. It is accepted that, in addition to a complete R0 resection, adjuvant therapy (administered before and/or after surgery) can significantly improve patients' outcomes. In Europe and the United States, a predominant approach is to administer perioperative chemotherapy for resectable gastroesophageal cancer, based on the Medical Research Council Adjuvant Gastric Infusional Chemotherapy (MAGIC) trial.[30] The MAGIC study was the first trial to show an improvement of survival by perioperative chemotherapy in patients with gastric, gastroesophageal junction (GEJ), and lower esophageal cancers. In this trial, the chemotherapy arm showed a statistically significant improvement in overall survival (OS) (5-year rates 36% vs 23%; hazard ratio [HR] 0.75; 95% CI, 0.60–0.93; $P = .009$) compared with surgery alone. A similar degree of benefit was noted in the second landmark trial of perioperative chemotherapy, the French Fédération Nationale des Centres de Lutte contre le Cancer (FNCLCC)/the Fédération Francophone de Cancérologie Digestive (FFCD) 9703 study.[31] Treatment with neoadjuvant or perioperative chemotherapy resulted in significantly improved OS (5-year OS rate 38% vs 24%; HR 0.69; 95% CI, 0.50–0.95; $P = .02$). Similar to the MAGIC trial, the subgroup of GEJ tumors derived the highest benefit from perioperative chemotherapy (HR 0.57; 95% CI, 0.39–0.83).

Studies from Asia have demonstrated the benefit of adjuvant therapy as well. The landmark studies include the Adjuvant capecitabine and oxaliplatin for gastric cancer after D2 gastrectomy (CLASSIC) study, which evaluated the role of adjuvant capecitabine and oxaliplatin in patients with resected gastric cancer[32] and adjuvant S-1.[33] In the adjuvant XELOX (capecitabine plus oxaliplatin) study (CLASSIC), adjuvant chemotherapy significantly improved disease-free survival: 3-year disease-free survival was 74% (95% CI, 69–79) in the chemotherapy and surgery group and 59% (53–64) in the surgery-only group (HR 0.56; 95% CI, 0.44–0.72; $P<.0001$).[32] Similarly, adjuvant S-1 also significantly improved patient outcomes: HR 0.68 (95% CI, 0.52–0.87; $P = .003$).[33]

Integration of Targeted Therapies

The integration of targeted therapy in the neoadjuvant/adjuvant setting is likely to hold the most promise above current standard approaches. Human epidermal growth factor receptor 2 (HER-2)–directed therapy improved survival in patients with metastatic HER-2–positive gastric and GEJ adnocarcinoma[34] and represents a promising predictive marker for HER-2–positive, early stage disease. However, the addition of HER-2–targeted therapy to chemotherapy in the neoadjuvant or adjuvant setting remains unproven and is being examined in Europe (NCT02581462, NCT02205047). These studies include the use of pertuzumab in addition to trastuzumab as the method of targeting HER-2 signaling.

The application of immunotherapy in the minimal residual disease setting is another exciting approach. As summarized in Drs Murphy and Kelly's article on "The Evolving Role of Checkpoint Inhibitors in the Management of Gastroesophageal Cancer," in this issue, the role of programmed cell death 1 (PD-1)/PD-L1 expression as a biomarker for efficacy of checkpoint inhibition remains controversial; there is evidence of its expression correlating with patient outcomes.[35,36] Ohigashi and colleagues[35] evaluated PD-L1 and PD-L2 gene expression in 41 esophagectomy patients by real-time quantitative polymerase chain reaction.[35] There was no significant relationship between either PD-L1 or PD-L2 expression and the age at surgery, sex, or pathologic stage, including nodal status. OS of patients with tumors positive for both PD-L1 and PD-L2 was significantly worse than that with tumors negative for both (50% vs 100% 1-year survival, $P = .0008$).[35] Kono and colleagues[36] also demonstrated that patients with esophagogastric cancer who had higher levels of regulatory T cells (which are CD4$^+$CD25^{high}), which inhibit the immune system, had poorer survival. Based on the initial exciting data of checkpoint inhibition in advanced disease settings, PD-1 inhibition is currently being tested in the adjuvant setting, with the hope of significantly improving patient survival (NCT02743494).

Application of Novel Imaging to Identify Response

A novel use of current imaging technology uses functional imaging as a radiographic biomarker of chemotherapy efficacy. Serial ^{18}F-2-fluoro-2-deoxyglucose (FDG)-PET/computed tomography scanning can identify response to preoperative chemotherapy by evaluation of the change from baseline in the standardized uptake value of the administered FDG. This response may be identified early in the preoperative treatment plan, before completion of the first cycle.[37–41] FDG-PET nonresponders, which comprise approximately 50% of patients who initiate preoperative therapy, have significantly worse outcomes. However, what do we do if we identify early that a patient is destined for a worse outcome? This question is being studied in a US national trial, asking the following question: Would early assessment of response afford the opportunity to modify therapy in those patients who are not responding in an effort to improve patient outcomes (NCT02485834)? The study, A021302: Impact of early FDG-PET directed intervention on preoperative therapy for locally advanced gastric cancer: a randomized phase 2 study, patients with FDG-avid locally advanced gastric cancer receive standard preoperative chemotherapy in cycle 1, attempts to answer this question. An on-study PET scan is performed at the end of cycle 1 to determine if patients are classified as a PET responder or PET nonresponder. PET nonresponders (about 50% of all patients) will then go on to enroll in the study if they remain surgical candidates, being randomized to salvage perioperative chemotherapy with docetaxel/irinotecan or to surgery followed by chemoradiation.

SUMMARY

It is apparent that as our advances in gastric and esophageal cancer come to fruition, we will begin to experience improvements in patient survival. Some of the key areas to impact on patient outcomes will be in understanding the molecular underpinnings of the onset of disease, the application of targeted therapies to disease subtypes, and the introduction of novel treatment paradigms in the locally advanced setting. Ultimately, by treating the right patients at the right time with the right therapies, we hope to transform our care of patients with gastric and esophageal cancer in hopes of improving survival far beyond its current state. To achieve these goals, the author anticipates an increasing number of clinical studies, which is our imperative to fulfill.

REFERENCES

1. Choi KS, Jun JK, Suh M, et al. Effect of endoscopy screening on stage at gastric cancer diagnosis: results of the National Cancer Screening Programme in Korea. Br J Cancer 2013;112(3):608–12.
2. Siegel R, Ma J, Zou Z, et al. Cancer statistics, 2014. CA Cancer J Clin 2014;64(1): 9–29.
3. Shah MA. Gastrointestinal cancer: targeted therapies in gastric cancer - the dawn of a new era. Nat Rev Clin Oncol 2014;11(1):10–1.
4. Power DG, Kelsen DP, Shah MA. Advanced gastric cancer - slow but steady progress. Cancer Treat Rev 2010;36(5):384–92.
5. Shah MA, Kelsen DP. Gastric cancer: a primer on the epidemiology and biology of the disease and an overview of the medical management of advanced disease. J Natl Compr Canc Netw 2010;8(4):437–47.
6. Ferlay J, Soerjomataram I, Dikshit R, et al. Cancer incidence and mortality worldwide: sources, methods and major patterns in GLOBOCAN 2012. Int J Cancer 2015;136(5):E359–86.
7. Jackson C, Cunningham D, Oliveira J, ESMO Guidelines Working Group, et al. Gastric cancer: ESMO clinical recommendations for diagnosis, treatment and follow-up. Ann Oncol 2009;20(Suppl 4):iv34–6.
8. Jemal A, Bray F, Center MM, et al. Global cancer statistics. CA Cancer J Clin 2011;61:69–90.
9. Shah MA, Khanin R, Tang L, et al. Molecular classification of gastric cancer: a new paradigm. Clin Cancer Res 2011;17(9):2693–701.
10. Fitzgerald RC, Hardwick R, Huntsman D, et al. Hereditary diffuse gastric cancer: updated consensus guidelines for clinical management and directions for future research. J Med Genet 2010;47(7):436–44.
11. Lynch HT, Grady W, Suriano G, et al. Gastric cancer: new genetic developments. J Surg Oncol 2005;90(3):114–33.
12. Huntsman DG, Carneiro F, Lewis FR, et al. Early gastric cancer in young, asymptomatic carriers of germ-line E-cadherin mutations. N Engl J Med 2001;344(25): 1904–9.
13. Crew KD, Neugut AI. Epidemiology of gastric cancer. World J Gastroenterol 2006;12(3):354–62.
14. Lichtenstein P, Holm NV, Verkasalo PK, et al. Environmental and heritable factors in the causation of cancer. N Engl J Med 2000;343(2):78–85.

15. Peek RMJ, Blaser MJ. Helicobacter pylori and gastrointestinal tract adenocarcinomas. Nat Rev Cancer 2002;2:28–37.
16. Schistosomes, liver flukes and Helicobacter pylori. IARC Working Group on the Evaluation of Carcinogenic Risks to Humans. Lyon, 7-14 June 1994. IARC Monogr Eval Carcinog Risks Hum 1994;61:1–241.
17. Uemura N, Okamoto S, Yamamoto S, et al. Helicobacter pylori infection and the development of gastric cancer. N Engl J Med 2001;345(11):784–9.
18. Correa P. Is gastric cancer preventable? Gut 2004;53(9):1217–9.
19. The Cancer Genome Atlas Research. Comprehensive molecular characterization of gastric adenocarcinoma. Nature 2014;513(7517):202–9.
20. Lie Z, Tan IB, Das K, et al. Identification of molecular subtypes of gastric cancer with different responses to PI3-Kinase inhibitors and 5-fluorouracil. Gastroenterology 2013;145(3):554–65.
21. Yun J, Mullarky E, Lu C, et al. Vitamin C selectively kills KRAS and BRAF mutant colorectal cancer cells by targeting GAPDH. Science 2015;350(6266):1391–6.
22. Tan P, Yeoh KG. Genetics and molecular pathogenesis of gastric adenocarcinoma. Gastroenterology 2015;149:1153–62.
23. Le DT, Uram JN, Wang H, et al. PD-1 blockade in tumors with mismatch-repair deficiency. N Engl J Med 2015;372(26):2509–20.
24. Hansford S, Kaurah P, Li-Chang H, et al. Hereditary diffuse gastric cancer syndrome: CDH1 mutations and beyond. JAMA Oncol 2015;1(1):23–32.
25. Antoniou AC, Casadei S, Heikkinen T, et al. Breast-cancer risk in families with mutations in PALB2. N Engl J Med 2014;371(6):497–506.
26. Bacani JT, Soares M, Zwingerman R, et al. CDH1/E-cadherin germline mutations in early-onset gastric cancer. J Med Genet 2006;43(11):867–72.
27. Benusiglio PR, Malka D, Rouleau E, et al. CDH1 germline mutations and the hereditary diffuse gastric and lobular breast cancer syndrome: a multicentre study. J Med Genet 2013;50(7):486–9.
28. Wang K, Yuen ST, Xu J, et al. Whole-genome sequencing and comprehensive molecular profiling identify new driver mutations in gastric cancer. Nat Genet 2014;46(6):573–82.
29. Yao F, Kausalya JP, Sia YY, et al. Recurrent fusion genes in gastric cancer: CLDN18-ARHGAP26 induces loss of epithelial integrity. Cell Rep 2015;12:272–85.
30. Cunningham D, Allum WH, Stenning SP, et al. Perioperative chemotherapy versus surgery alone for resectable gastroesophageal cancer. N Engl J Med 2006;355(1):11–20.
31. Ychou M, Boige V, Pignon JP, et al. Perioperative chemotherapy compared with surgery alone for resectable gastroesophageal adenocarcinoma: an FNCLCC and FFCD multicenter phase III trial. J Clin Oncol 2011;29(13):1715–21.
32. Bang YJ, Kim YW, Yang HK, et al. Adjuvant capecitabine and oxaliplatin for gastric cancer after D2 gastrectomy (CLASSIC): a phase 3 open-label, randomised controlled trial. Lancet 2012;379(9813):315–21.
33. Sakuramoto S, Sasako M, Yamaguchi T, et al. Adjuvant chemotherapy for gastric cancer with S-1, an oral fluoropyrimidine. N Engl J Med 2007;357(18):1810–20.
34. Bang YJ, Van Cutsem E, Feyereislova A, et al. Trastuzumab in combination with chemotherapy versus chemotherapy alone for treatment of HER2-positive advanced gastric or gastro-oesophageal junction cancer (ToGA): a phase 3, open-label, randomised controlled trial. Lancet 2010;376(9742):687–97.

35. Ohigashi Y, Sho M, Yamada Y, et al. Clinical significance of programmed death-1 ligand-1 and programmed death-1 ligand-2 expression in human esophageal cancer. Clin Cancer Res 2005;11(8):2947–53.

36. Kono K, Kawaida H, Takahashi A, et al. CD4(+)CD25high regulatory T cells increase with tumor stage in patients with gastric and esophageal cancers. Cancer Immunol Immunother 2006;55(9):1064–71.

37. Wieder HA, Brücher BL, Zimmermann F, et al. Time course of tumor metabolic activity during chemoradiotherapy of esophageal squamous cell carcinoma and response to treatment. J Clin Oncol 2004;22(5):900–8.

38. Ott K, Weber WA, Lordick F, et al. Metabolic imaging predicts response, survival, and recurrence in adenocarcinomas of the esophagogastric junction. J Clin Oncol 2006;24(29):4692–8.

39. Lordick F, Ott K, Krause BJ, et al. PET to assess early metabolic response and to guide treatment of adenocarcinoma of the oesophagogastric junction: the MUNICON phase II trial. Lancet Oncol 2007;8(9):797–805.

40. Ott K, Herrmann K, Lordick F, et al. Early metabolic response evaluation by fluorine-18 fluorodeoxyglucose positron emission tomography allows in vivo testing of chemosensitivity in gastric cancer: long-term results of a prospective study. Clin Cancer Res 2008;14(7):2012–8.

41. Shah MA, Yeung H, Coit D, et al. A phase II study of preoperative chemotherapy with irinotecan (CPT) and cisplatin (CIS) for gastric cancer(NCI 5917): FDG-PET/CT predicts patient outcome. Orlando (FL): American Society of Clinical Oncology, Annual Proceedings; 2007 [abstract: 4502].

Index

Note: Page numbers of article titles are in **boldface** type.

Hematol Oncol Clin N Am 31 (2017) 553–563
http://dx.doi.org/10.1016/S0889-8588(17)30045-X
0889-8588/17

hemonc.theclinics.com